ISOME

The simplest way to incre muscle tone. Includes fitness programmes for men and for women, isometrics for the bed-bound and disabled, and a special series of exercises for those wishing to gain maximum strength and power.

ISOMETRICS

The Short Cut to Fitness

by

**James
Hewitt**

THORSONS PUBLISHERS LIMITED
Wellingborough, Northamptonshire

First published 1980
Second Impression 1981

British Library Cataloguing in Publication Data

Hewitt, James
    Isometrics.
    1. Isometric exercise
    I. Title
    613.7'1   RA781.2

    ISBN 0-7225-0604-X

Printed in Great Britain by
King's English Bookprinters Limited, Bramley, Leeds,
and bound by Weatherby Woolnough,
Wellingborough, Northamptonshire.

Contents

1.

What is Isometrics?

Isometrics, or isometric contraction exercise, is a physical fitness method that is invaluable for the man or woman who welcomes a short cut to improved muscle strength, shape and tone. It is the nearest thing you can find to instant exercise. Even if it is not as effortless as pouring boiling water onto coffee powder, it is certainly, as a physical performance, just as simple. It is literally as simple as pressing the palms of your hands together – which is a good example of this kind of exercise.

Isometric exercises are static muscle contractions produced by exerting steady pressure in held positions without moving your limbs – not even a little. There are no problems about your not being strong enough, supple enough, or clever enough. Everybody can practise isometrics. Each contraction lasts only a few seconds, so there is no endurance problem. To exercise you need only the space you stand in. A programme takes only a few minutes, even when you include rest pauses between contractions. Yet it can produce valuable results in improved health, fitness and appearance.

As a physical fitness system, isometrics has other advantages. You do not need special clothing, neither do you need to join a club, pay membership fees or to have an instructor. A book can teach you what you need to know about effective practice. The demand on your time and will-power is slight and it requires no special equipment or apparatus: ordinary household fixtures and furniture may be utilized, but mostly you pit one part of your body against another part to produce contractions.

In view of these many advantages as a home-exercise system, it is not surprising that the first systematized use of isometrics for enhancing physical fitness should have been accompanied by considerable publicity. Non-movement exercise was an exciting new concept.

People with interests in vigorous physical activity have a special reason for using isometrics, since increased muscle strength and tone will improve performance in athletics, sports and games. But it is just as useful for people in all walks of life who do not go in for vigorous leisure pursuits. Men, women and children benefit. People of all ages can practise it.

However, it is not suitable for people who have heart disease, high blood pressure, and perhaps some other health problems. Injuries and weaknesses may preclude contractions for certain areas of the body, though isometrics has a role in the rehabilitation of the injured. Any reader who has doubts about the suitability of performing isometric contractions because of some physical injury or health problem should take the advice of a doctor on whether or not isometrics would be harmful. For the majority of people, however, practice is possible and highly beneficial.

Programmes for All

In this book there are programmes of isometric contraction exercises to suit all needs. Those for men and for women allow for moderate, average and maximum strength requirements. There is a programme for the person seeking great muscular strength, whether for its own sake or for improvement in athletics, sports or games. Advice is given on how to use isometric contractions to improve strength and tone in the muscles most used in an activity. There is a programme that can be practised while seated, and one that can be performed while lying in bed. In another section advice is given on how a programme may be shared with a partner.

All these programmes contract muscles from head to feet. Planned exercise of this kind exercises the whole body systematically, something which is not done by sports and games. In many sports and games there is an over-emphasis on the use of certain parts of the body.

Scientific Research

Isometrics is an exercise method based on scientific research. It became a physical culture 'craze' in the USA in the early 1960s following research by Dr T. Hettinger. He had systematically explored the effects of static muscle contractions at the Max Planck Institute in Dortmund and later at the Lankenau Hospital in Philadelphia. In one experiment, one leg of a frog was tied and its other leg was left free. The leg that was tied gained considerably in strength because the frog had tugged against the bond; the frog had in fact engaged in isometric contraction exercise.

Hettinger showed why isometrics produces a rapid increase in muscle strength and tone. In most muscle activity only a minority of muscle fibres are contracted, but when a muscle is pitted against an immovable object the result is a static contraction of *all* the muscle fibres. If at least two-thirds of a person's maximum strength is used, static contraction exercise will produce a rapid increase in strength.

While the main reasons for such research was connected with the rehabilitation of certain hospital patients, physical culturists were not slow to see the importance of Hettinger's findings. Athletes, footballers and other sportsmen were soon using isometric contractions in their training.

Isometric and Isotonic

Exercise, as most people understand it, is linked with movement of the limbs and with shortening and lengthening of body muscles. This is isotonic muscle activity. The word isotonic means equal tones or equal tension. Examples of this kind of muscle work are found in sports, athletics, weight-training, gymnastics, calisthenics, cycling, swimming, and so on. Regular, active exercise makes an essential contribution to maintaining physical fitness. This is exercise as the proverbial man on a Clapham omnibus understands it. Isometric exercise is not so well known.

There is no necessity here to go deeply into the functioning of muscles, but the following information is worth noting. Muscle fibres respond to nervous stimulus in one of three ways:

1. They shorten, for example, when raising an arm or a leg. This is called *concentric* muscle work.
2. They lengthen, as in slowly lowering an arm or a leg. This is *eccentric* muscle work. (If an arm or a leg is brought down faster than gravity would achieve, certain muscles work concentrically to produce the fast pull).
3. They neither shorten nor lengthen, but hold a fixed position. This is static or *isometric* muscle activity. The word means 'same length'.

Concentric and eccentric muscle work are examples of isotonic muscle activity. If you find the word isometric too technical, think of static instead.

You are probably very familiar with exercise as movement,

but note that you use your muscles isometrically every day in staying erect. As a popular system of physical exercise isometrics is of recent origin, but that is not to say static contractions were not part of some forms of exercise before the fuss about isometrics arose in the USA. The most venerable body-culture system still in use – and much in use in the West today – is that of Hatha Yoga, whose origins go back more than two thousand years. Its postures are held without movement and many involve the isometric contraction of muscles. We will include some in the programmes given in this book. The *Sandow Magazine* for July 1898 contained a programme of static contractions under the heading 'Physical Culture Without Exercise'. Sandow was the most famous muscle-man of the Victorian period.

If you think of exercise as movement, then isometrics could seem to be 'physical culture without exercise'. It may be looked upon as movement exercise frozen at some point. The attempted movement should be against resistance. No special equipment is necessary. One part of your body can block the movement of another part or you can find an immovable object to provide an unyielding resistance. A wall will do, or a door, or a door frame, or a table or desk. You do not move your limbs, but you exert strong pressure which produces a static or isometric contraction of the muscle fibres. What are the benefits?

More Strength and Energy

Essentially isometrics is a way to build strength and improve muscle tone through static contractions of the skeletal muscles. The body being a unit, exercise of the skeletal muscles benefits the whole human organism. Fatigue is reduced and efficiency is increased. The body builds up defences against disease and stress. The aches and pains that plague some lives are dispersed.

Every person benefits from having energy and strength beyond normal requirements. With this reserve capital, you will not be put under sudden strain when called on to exert unaccustomed muscular effort – pushing a car, shovelling snow, digging a garden, and so on. This kind of exertion is responsible for many heart attacks. Physical fitness will protect your heart. There is also the possibility of having to cope with an unexpected emergency on which your life or that of a loved one may depend. There is also the psychological importance of knowing that you have strength in reserve. You will feel happier and more secure for knowing that you are living on the interest of your energy capital and that reserves of strength are there when needed.

If you practise daily any of the programmes given in this book, you will soon find that your energy and strength are increasing. It is like depositing money in a bank account. Strength and energy are forms of wealth, and among the finest there is. George Bernard Shaw, in explaining economics to the intelligent woman, concisely defined capital as 'money to spare'. Having strength and energy to spare is the secret of the 'first wealth' which is health.

Improved Muscle Tone

Exercise of the skeletal muscles improves their tone. Muscle tone has two meanings. One meaning is the overall health of a muscle: its strength, firmness, texture and elasticity. Another meaning of muscle tone is the subtle contraction which keeps a skeletal muscle in a state of constant readiness for action. Partial muscle contraction also keeps the body from collapsing through lack of support. As mentioned earlier, isometric contractions play an essential role in keeping the body upright. The skeletal muscles of the fit person respond rapidly and efficiently to commands from the brain.

Incidentally, a similar tonus seems also to be necessary for health of the psyche. Dr Viktor E. Frankl, the existentialist psychologist, writes in *Man's Search for Meaning* '... mental health is based on a certain degree of tension, the tension between what one has already achieved and what one still ought to accomplish, or the gap between what one is and what one should become. Such a tension is inherent in the human being and therefore is indispensable to mental well-being.' There is also a kind of mental tonus called intentionality, whereby we grasp life and find it meaningful. It is the experience of most people that good muscle tone is propitious to good mental tone.

Efficiency and Effectiveness

Improved physical strength and fitness is manifested in greater efficiency and effectiveness in life's varied activities; whether it be ascending a flight of stairs or steps, turning over soil in the garden, shopping, pushing a pram, carrying a child, carrying suitcases, playing with children, shovelling snow, jogging, or hurrying to catch a bus or train. Work productivity is likely to be enhanced, whether your job is markedly physical or not. I have already pointed out the link between body fitness and the quality of consciousness.

Improvement in Sports and Athletics
Greater strength and improved muscle tone make for greater success in sports and athletics. Isometrics has been incorporated into the training of top athletes, footballers and tennis professionals. Coaches were among the first people to recognize its potential. USA Olympic weight-lifting coach, Bob Hoffman, exclaimed: 'I am absolutely awestruck by the miracles it has wrought. Let's make full use of this great gift from heaven!'

If you wish to improve your performance in any athletic event, sport or game, get a clear grasp of the simple principle of isometric contraction exercise and apply it to your activity in the way described in the chapter 'Programme for Muscle Power'.

Improved Appearance
Bone structure cannot be altered and heredity determines to a basic extent the appearance of the human figure. But through exercise and obeying the rules of healthy living each of us can make the most of our bodies in the way of keeping their appearances youthful and pleasant to the eyes. Exercise builds muscle for the thin; flesh can be added in those places where it is most needed. It also removes fat that has accumulated in the wrong places. Even the face can be exercised, as a later chapter will show. Facial isometrics can make men and women look years younger.

The great number of unshapely bodies to be seen on the beaches of popular seaside resorts any summer cannot be blamed on heredity. They could be reshaped on more attractive lines through planned exercise and dietary control. If your problem is obesity, isometrics should be supported by restriction of the sugars and starches whose consumption has increased rapidly in the diet of the people of the more affluent nations. Refined sugar, white bread, white rice, jam, cakes and so on are high in calories – but they are 'empty' calories, supplying energy but lacking important minerals and vitamins or body-building and body-repairing nutrients.

It is instinctive good sense to want to look healthy and in good physical shape and condition. About thirty years ago I purchased a little book called *Psychology for Everyman (and Woman)*, written by A.E. Mander. In plain language it explains human behaviour. The author lists thirteen primary human wants. In an earlier book, that is now out of print, I gave a commentary showing how each of the thirteen human needs are satisfied in some way by having a strong and shapely body. Space does not allow a similar commentary here, but readers should be able to see for themselves the relevance of physical fitness to each need. The thirteen wants:

1. For bodily comfort.
2. For a sense of security.
3. To escape.
4. To propitiate anyone who has power to injure; to ingratiate oneself.
5. To be noticed, admired and liked by others of one's kind.
6. To hurt and injure, to overcome and dominate, to feel superior.
7. To attract, please and mate with one of the opposite sex.
8. To look after and protect someone (eg child or mate) who is relatively weak.
9. For the company and fellow-feeling of others of one's kind.
10. To be like others of one's own 'pack' or 'set', especially its leaders.
11. To catch and capture.
12. To find out, to know, to understand.
13. To return to familiar people, places, and conditions.

For 13 I will repeat my earlier commentary: 'To return to one's true animal muscularity and natural body/mind integration following years of neglect and alienation is to "return home" at a deep instinctive level.'

Increased Fitness

The benefits of the practice of isometrics stated above may be summed up in two words – increased fitness. How should we define 'fitness'? The definition I have in mind is one that can be a comfortable target for the average man or woman. It was given by Dr Warren Redwood Guild in his book *How to Keep Fit and Enjoy It*: 'Adequate fitness allows the individual to perform his daily chores without interference by fatigue, to have sufficient physical reserve to meet unexpected emergencies safely, and to have enough extra energy to enjoy leisure time.' As you can see, fitness is that strength and energy to spare or health capital which I discussed earlier.

2.

General Rules for Practice

This chapter gives general rules for the practice of isometrics. Where there are exceptions to the general rules or slight variations, these will be indicated in the introduction to a programme or in the description of one of the contractions. Rules for specific programmes will be given before describing the programme.

Who?

Almost everyone can practise isometrics. The contractions are based on held positions which are simple to adopt: you then exert pressure without movement. There are no problems of insufficient strength, skill, or suppleness. This means that men and women of all ages can strengthen, firm, tone, and shape their muscles by this method.

As strong sustained pressure is used for some seconds, the method may be dangerous for people with weak hearts or high blood pressure. People with serious health problems should ask a doctor whether or not they could safely practise isometrics. It is a sound precaution for middle-aged or older people to receive a doctor's permission to practise.

When?

Any time of day will do to perform an isometric programme, but most people get into the habit of setting aside the few minutes required at a fixed time each day. If you exercise in the morning before breakfast, warm up for a minute or two with easy movements before starting the contractions, to give your muscles the chance to 'awaken'. Allow an hour or more to pass after a light meal and two hours after your main meal of the day. If an isometric programme is practised shortly before an evening meal, it seems to squeeze away the fatigues and toxins of the working day. Also, most people find they do not overeat after exercise, which could be useful for the man or woman inclined to put on excess weight. Other people prefer to exercise just before going to bed, and they say they sink rapidly into sound sleep.

The choice of time of day is yours. Best results come from daily practice, but if your strength aims are moderate every other day may be satisfactory.

Where?

Most people perform isometrics at home and at a particular time of day. A few people exercise in an office, making use for some contractions of desks, filing cabinets, typewriters, and so on to provide unyielding resistance to pressure. Similarly, home furniture, walls, doors, and so on may be used as aids. For most exercises all the space you need is that which you stand or sit in. Contractions may be improvised as you wait in a car in a traffic jam or on some other occasion seized as a fitness opportunity. However, these are additional contractions and should not be substituted for your regular programme.

Clothing

No special clothing is required. Temperature and other circumstances permitting, the less clothing you wear the better. Underpants for men and panties and bra for women give maximum comfort and freedom.

How?

Isometric contractions are static muscle contractions produced by exerting pressure against an immovable and unyielding object. The result may come through one part of your body blocking an attempt at movement by another part, as in trying to turn your head to right or left and blocking any movement with counter pressure from your right or left hand respectively. The immovable object may be a door, wall, table, post, or even another part of your own body. Pressure for six to fifteen seconds produces a muscle contraction which strengthens and tones the muscle even though there is no movement.

In movement or isotonic exercise your muscles shorten or lengthen as your body moves. In isometrics the muscle fibres contract but are not worked over their range of movement. If you think of isometric exercises as checked movements, which most of them are in the programmes to follow, then one example will illustrate clearly the principle of the 'held position' in isometrics.

One way to exercise the biceps brachi at the front of the upper arm is to make it perform its normal function of flexing the arm, but against resistance. In weight-training the resistance would come from a bar-bell which is held at shoulders' width and at arms' length across the tops of the thighs and is then 'curled' up to the shoulders. The weight is slowly brought up and lowered perhaps fifteen times. As the arms become stronger, more weight is added to the bar-bell. The biceps shorten in raising the bar and lengthen in lowering it.

The same exercise is performed *isometrically* by holding your arms partly flexed and trying to complete the flexion but preventing any movement by blocking it with the aid of a table or desk or pitting one arm against the other. (See contractions M6A and P6A.)

Other exercises are based on held positions where the action seems to have been 'frozen' at some point by blocking it. The principle is simple. Your body still needs movement exercise (see the final chapter) – but isometrics has obvious advantages as a speedy method of improving muscle strength and tone.

Breathing During Contractions

Before each contraction, take a deep and comfortable breath, unless otherwise instructed. Draw air deep down, as though into your abdomen as well as expanding your chest. Breathe in and out through your nostrils unless they are blocked or the special nature of the exercise requires breathing through the mouth. Most people will find they can take a breath then release it slowly during a contraction lasting eight to ten seconds. Some people find that the slow release of air following the initial inhalation can continue comfortably for the whole of the contraction, even when of maximum duration of fifteen seconds. Avoid discomfort or strain in your breathing: take an extra breath if you really need it, but remember that unnecessary inhalations disrupt momentarily the steadiness of your pressure.

A few contractions of a special nature require performance on emptied lungs and suspended breathing: their duration has been kept down to six seconds, which is comfortable. Normally you should not hold your breath during contractions.

Force and Duration of Contraction

The number of seconds each contraction is sustained and the degree of strength exerted depends on how much strength is sought. I have allowed for three categories of strength-seekers.

The first category has moderate or mild strength requirements. Most women and most men over forty (and some under) will fit into this category. They seek a secure level of strength and fitness but without taxing their strength in exercise to near maximum or maximum. You start by exerting half maximum strength in the first week and then increasing pressure during the second week to two-thirds or three-quarters of maximum strength. The duration of each contraction starts at six seconds and increases a second a week to ten seconds.

The second category of strength seeker I call 'standard' for want of a better word. This is the category that the majority of men under thirty probably belong in. Here the aim is for a near maximum gain in strength and about ninety per cent of maximum strength is exerted in each contraction. The duration of each contraction starts at six seconds and increases to twelve seconds.

The third category is for the dedicated body-builder, weight-lifter, athlete, sportsman and sportswoman, seeking a maximum strength increase. Research shows that maximum results are obtained by exerting maximum strength for a contraction lasting fifteen seconds. A paper by Helen J. Hislop published in the *Journal of the American Physical Therapy Association* reported gains of over twenty per cent increase of strength in the left bicep muscle over a training period of seven weeks through contracting the muscle twice daily at maximum strength for fifteen seconds. Start at nine seconds and add one second a week until reaching fifteen seconds.

Whatever your category, always apply steady pressure. You will risk muscle strain if you start off with a snap or a jerk. Stiffness can be avoided or kept slight if for the first week you apply pressure a little below what your category demands. Slight stiffness soon clears. Take thirty to sixty seconds rest between contractions.

Keeping a Progress Chart

Improvements in weight gain or weight loss and in body measurements may be recorded. The specimen chart shown may be used for the first five months of training, or you may prefer to copy the wording into a notebook. Weigh and measure on the first day of each month or on the same day of each month.

Use a reliable weighing machine, preferably always the same one. Wear the same weight of clothing each time or no clothing at all. Weigh yourself at the same hour of the day as body-weight fluctuates during the day. A good time is first thing in the morning after emptying the bladder.

In measuring your neck, chest, arms, hips, thighs, and calves, place the tape around the broadest part. In measuring your waist, place the tape around the narrowest part. In measuring your normal chest or bust, stand upright, your head level, your arms by your sides, with no exaggerated thrusting forward of the chest. Place the tape across the nipples and below the arm-pits. Men may measure the upper arm flexed and women with the arm straight.

PROGRESS CHART

	Before Starting	After 4 Weeks	After 8 Weeks	After 12 Weeks	After 16 Weeks	After 20 Weeks
Weight						
Neck						
Chest (bust)						
Upper arm						
Waist						
Hips						
Thigh						
Calf						

3.

Programme for Men

Isometric contractions firm and reshape the body, producing a more impressive, a more athletic and a more youthful appearance. All men will welcome this. They also build and maintain muscular strength.

How much strength does modern man need? The answer is that individual needs will vary according to occupation, age, and whether or not a man wishes to excel in athletics and in sports and games. The question arises because modern man is no longer a hunter like his primitive ancestors – running, fighting, lifting, dragging, killing to provide food and clothing for himself and his family – and because his work (with exceptions) has been mechanized to the point where little physical exertion is needed to earn a living. But even the sedentary worker requires an optimal standard of muscular strength and tone for efficient and healthy living. The advances of modern technology have meant that millions of men are denying their bodies adequate exercise for health. Additional hazards arise from the greatly increased consumption of sugars and starches in the modern diet. Doctors warn that the combination of inadequate exercise and overweight are responsible for a build up of fatty substances in the blood and the lining of the arteries in men that leads to heart attacks and numerous deaths.

The case for having sufficient energy and strength to act as reserve capital has been stated earlier. Such a reserve is protection against stress, that great modern killer, and it fosters health and self-confidence.

Many men feel an instinctive need for muscular strength. Male muscularity cries out to be used. Male inactivity, flabbiness and feebleness are often accompanied by feelings of guilt, whether conscious or unconscious. Redressing the 'wrong' by building a firm strong body is correspondingly accompanied by feelings of confidence and well-being. These factors are deep-rooted in the nature and history of man.

By long tradition many men equate muscular strength with masculinity. Other men seek muscular strength and tone for greater effectiveness in sports, games and athletics. Isometric contraction exercises have been incorporated in the training programmes of the US Marine Corps and those of the fighting men of other countries. It has also become part of the training programmes of Olympic athletes, footballers, swimmers, and enthusiasts for other sports.

The varying strength requirements of male readers of this book are taken into consideration in the instructions given below for the duration and performance of the contractions. Men desiring great strength for sports and athletics or for its own sake should practise the programme for men for four to six weeks to condition their muscles to static contractions and then move on to the programme for muscular power.

Instructions for Practice
General rules for practice were given in Chapter 2. The following points are worth noting again as they apply to the practice of the programme for men.

Breathing
Take a deep *comfortable* breath before starting the contraction. Feel as though the air is going down to your abdomen as well as expanding your chest. Breathe in and out through your nostrils unless they are blocked or the special nature of an exercise requires mouth breathing. Most men will find that if a deep breath is taken the air can be released slowly from the lungs during a contraction lasting up to ten seconds. A quick breath may then be taken and released slowly until the contraction is completed. However, some men will find that the slow release of air following the first inhalation can continue comfortably for the maximum duration of a contraction, which is fifteen seconds. The important thing is to avoid discomfort or strain in your breathing. Take an extra breath if you really need it, but remember that unnecessary inhalations disrupt momentarily the steadiness of your pressure.

Force and Duration of Contraction
Category A (moderate strength requirements). Begin by sustaining each contraction for five seconds (a slow count of one, two, three, four, five). Add one second to the duration of

each contraction at the end of each week until the duration of each contraction is ten seconds. Exert strong pressure without straining: about three-quarters of your maximum strength.

Category B (standard strength requirements). Begin by sustaining each contraction for six seconds (a slow count of one, two, three, four, five, six). Add one second per week until the duration of each contraction is twelve seconds. Exert powerful pressure, that is about ninety per cent of your maximum strength.

Category C (maximum strength requirements). Begin by sustaining each contraction for nine seconds. Add one second per week until the duration of each contraction is fifteen seconds. Exert maximum pressure.

All categories. To avoid muscle strain, do not start with a sudden jerk. Apply steady pressure.

M1A. Brow Clasp

Held Position
Stand upright, your back comfortably straight, your head poised on top of your spine, your chin parallel to the floor or ground, your eyes looking straight ahead without staring. Spread your legs a little apart to provide a firm base. This is the correct relaxed posture to adopt at the start of any standing isometric contraction exercise. Now interlock your fingers and place the palms of your clasped hands horizontally across your forehead. Hold out your elbows to full width level with your ears. Your back and head should form a straight vertical line without rigidity.

Contraction
Take a deep breath, expanding your chest, then PRESS YOUR HEAD FORWARD STRONGLY, BUT, AT THE SAME TIME, PREVENT ANY MOVEMENT OF THE HEAD OR BODY BY PRESSING BACKWARD WITH YOUR HANDS.

Purpose
To strengthen, firm, tone and shape the muscles of the neck. A scraggy neck is one of the first signs of advancing years. These three neck contractions will round out the neck and delay signs of ageing. In the Brow Clasp the chief muscles exercised are those at the front of the neck which thrust the head forward. As well as giving fullness to the neck, these

contractions improve posture by giving strong support for the head, a not inconsiderable weight to carry on top of the spine during the course of a day.

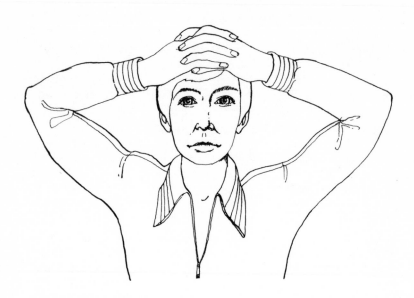

M1B. Head Clasp

Held Position
Stand relaxed and upright as for M1A, but now take your interlocked hands over your head and place the palms of your hands horizontally across the base of your skull, your elbows held out wide.

Contraction
Take a deep breath, expanding your chest, then PRESS YOUR HEAD BACKWARD STRONGLY BUT, AT THE SAME TIME, PREVENT ANY MOVEMENT OF THE HEAD OR BODY BY PRESSING FORWARD WITH YOUR HANDS. (See W1B for illustration).

Purpose
To strengthen, firm, tone and shape the muscles of the neck. In the Head Clasp the chief muscles exercised are those at the back of the neck which thrust the head backwards.

M1C. Head Turn

Held Position
Stand as for the start of M1A and M1B, that is, comfortably erect. Place the palm of your right hand horizontally across your right temple just above the ear. Raise your right elbow out wide to the side. Your fingers point towards the back of your head.

Contraction
Take a deep breath, expanding your chest. Keeping your head level and avoiding staring, ATTEMPT TO TURN YOUR HEAD TO THE RIGHT. BLOCK ANY MOVEMENT WITH COUNTER PRESSURE FROM YOUR RIGHT HAND AND ARM. Following the contraction, rest a few moments then REPEAT TO THE LEFT SIDE. The palm of the left hand is placed horizontally across the left temple, just above the left ear, and blocks an attempt to turn your head to the left.

Purpose
To strengthen, firm, tone and shape the muscles of the neck. In the Head Turn the chief muscles exercised are those of the right and left sides of the neck respectively, responsible for turning the head to the sides. The main muscle involved is the sterno-mastoid. In all three neck contraction exercises – M1A, M1B and M1C – the hands, wrists, forearms, upper arms, and shoulders are exercised to some extent.

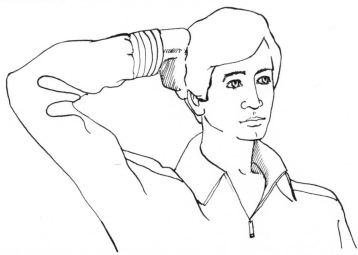

M2. Bent Arms Press In

Held Position

This is a simple exercise in which one arm competes with the
other arm in a trial of strength and the result should be a draw
for the duration of the contest. Stand comfortably erect,
looking straight ahead, your feet a little apart for firm support.
Bring the palms of your hands together in front of your chest,
your thumbs crossed. Grip firmly. The gesture is somewhat
similar to that indicating the receipt of joyous news. Raise
your elbows until your forearms are parallel to the floor or
ground. Your upper and lower arms should form a right
angle.

Contraction

Take a deep breath, expanding and raising your chest, then
PRESS YOUR HANDS TOGETHER STRONGLY. Exert
equal pressure from both arms so that your hands stay in one
position in front of your chest.

Purpose

To expand the chest and to strengthen, firm, tone and shape
the muscles of the chest, shoulders, and arms. The large
pectoral muscles of the chest will be seen to contract, if you
glance down or observe your reflection in a mirror.

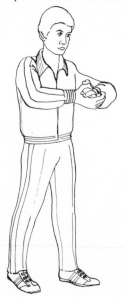

A variation of the Bent Arms Press In is to press your hands together directly overhead, holding your elbows out wide. This contracts the chest muscles in their upper fibres and also works the arms and shoulders from a different angle to the contraction, with the arms in front of the chest. This exercise is described in more detail in the Programme for Women W2.

M3. Bent Arms Pull Apart

Held Position
This may be looked upon as the converse of the preceding contraction M2, in which your hands were pressed together strongly with your arms bent. Now you link fingers and try to pull your hands apart. Stand upright, your feet a little apart. Again bring your hands together in front of your chest so that your upper and lower arms form right angles. But this time bend your fingers at their first and second joints and interlock the finger tips. Tuck your thumbs in for added resistance. Keep your elbows out so that the undersides of the arms are parallel to the floor or to the ground.

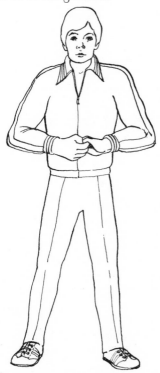

Contraction
Take a deep breath, expanding and raising your chest.
Looking straight ahead, TRY TO PULL YOUR HANDS
APART. If the fingers and thumbs are firmly interlocked,
neither arm should be able to claim victory and your hands
should stay in the same position. Stand perfectly still
throughout the contraction. It does not matter which hand is
nearest to you, the right or the left.

Purpose
To strengthen, firm, tone and shape the muscles of the
shoulder girdle and of the rear upper arms. The chief muscles
exercised are the deltoids, the trapezius, and the triceps.
    There is a variation that is the converse of that described for
the Bent Arms Press In. Link fingers directly overhead,
holding your elbows out wide and keeping your arms bent.
Try to pull your hands apart. This works the arms and
shoulders from a different angle.

M4. Overhead Pull Out

Held Position
Stand upright, looking straight ahead, your feet spread a little
apart to provide a strong base. Keep your weight distributed
evenly over both feet. Extend your arms to full length
overhead and pull a belt or a folded towel taut between your
hands (palms forward) to the same width as your shoulders.
Your arms will then be extended vertically.

Contraction
Take a deep breath, expanding your chest, then PULL
POWERFULLY OUTWARDS WITH YOUR HANDS as
though to tear the belt or towel apart.

Purpose
To strengthen, firm, tone and shape the muscles of the arms,
chest, shoulders, and upper back, and to improve posture.
The muscles of the upper back, in particular, are exercised in
this contraction.

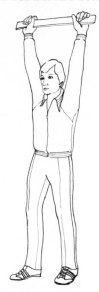

M5A. Finger Strengthening

A few seconds given daily to exercising your fingers and your grip will be repaid by giving you strong hands right into advanced years.

Stretch and spread your fingers and then press down your finger and thumb pads of both hands on a table or desk top or any other firm unyielding surface. You can liken it, if you wish, to giving a set of finger and thumb prints, or – a more pleasant image – to lingering over an emphatic chord you have just played on a grand piano.

Purpose
To strengthen the fingers and thumbs of both hands and to stimulate the circulation of blood in the hands.

M5B. Grip Strengthening

Athletes, sportsmen and sportswomen have a special interest in cultivating a strong grip. It is also helpful in certain occupations. But everybody benefits. Strong hands, hands which have power in reserve, conserve energy and make strength available for the kind of emergency on which life itself may depend. Weak hands in old age can be an irritation and an embarrassment and the following exercises will help you retain power in your grip.

The grip exercise is simple. Squeeze a hard ball – of the kind that children may play with or that dogs like to chew up.

A tennis ball may be used. Take a deep breath, then SQUEEZE IN STRONGLY, first with one hand and then with the other hand. If no ball is available, make fists of your hands and squeeze them hard, making your knuckles show white. This, too, is an isometric contraction. However, a suitable ball is worth setting aside for this daily exercise.

For a variation, try this. Hold a brush shaft or pole vertically before your chest. Bend your arms and grip the wood with the right hand immediately above the left, the hands touching. Twist the right hand in an anti-clockwise direction and twist the left hand in a clockwise direction. Rest a few seconds then repeat, exerting pressure with each hand in the reverse direction: clockwise with the right hand and anti-clockwise with the left hand. (If you are left-handed, place the left hand on top and the right hand beneath.)

Purpose
To strengthen your fingers, your grip, your wrists and your forearms.

M6A. Front Upper Arm Contraction

Held Position
The biceps muscle at the front of the upper arm has long been a symbol of manly strength. It helps flex the arm and is developed by flexing the arm against resistance, as in weight-training or, as here, in isometrics, by pitting the strength of one arm against the resistance of the other arm.

In showing the differences between isotonic and isometric exercises, I described the weight-training exercise known as 'the curl'. A bar-bell is held at arms' length across the thighs, at shoulders' width, palms upwards. The elbows are kept in against the sides. Keeping the body upright and the upper arms steady, the bar-bell is slowly 'curled' up, flexing the arms, to the chest. It is helpful to hold an image of this exercise when performing the isometric contraction described here.

As usual, the isometric exercise is a frustrated attempt at a movement exercise. Stand erect, your head and back in a vertical line, looking straight ahead and spreading your feet a little apart to aid good balance. The held position is with the arms flexed about half-way in what might have been the bar-bell or dumb-bell movement. Upper and lower arms form right angles. Your upper arms and elbows should be in contact with your sides. The best image is of a single arm dumb-bell 'curl', for here we contract each bicep separately, resisting with the other arm.

Flex your right arm to form a right angle between upper and lower arm. Your upper arm and elbow should be in contact with your right side. Now bring your left hand and forearm across your diaphragm. Form a fist with your left hand, thumb upwards, and rest it lightly on the palm of your right hand.

Contraction

Take a deep breath, expanding and raising your chest. PRESS YOUR LEFT FIST DOWN HARD ON YOUR RIGHT HAND AND, AT THE SAME TIME, TRY HARD TO BRING UP YOUR RIGHT HAND AS THOUGH TO COMPLETE THE SECOND HALF OF THE 'CURL' EXERCISE. Though there should be no movement, the biceps will contract strongly, just as it would in the dumb-bell exercise. Rest a few moments then REPEAT, REVERSING THE HAND AND ARM POSITIONS AND ATTEMPTING TO COMPLETE THE FLEXION OF THE LEFT ARM.

Purpose
To strengthen, firm, tone and shape the muscles of the arms, concentrating on the biceps muscle at the front of the upper arm. In the arm resisting flexion it will be the triceps muscle, the antagonist of the biceps, that is chiefly exercised.

M6B. Rear Upper Arm Contraction

Held Position
To concentrate more directly on the triceps at the rear of your upper arm, you have only to reverse the positions taken by your hands in the preceding biceps exercise. Now instead of attempting to complete the flexion of your arm you attempt to extend and straighten it against resistance from your other arm.

Again your right arm is bent to form a right angle between your upper and lower arm, your elbow and upper arm are held in against your ribs, and the palm of your right hand is turned upward. Now make a fist of your right hand. Bring your left arm across your body and place the palm of your left hand *under* your right fist.

Contraction
Take a deep breath, expanding and raising your chest, then PRESS DOWN STRONGLY WITH YOUR RIGHT FIST AND AT THE SAME TIME PRESS UP STRONGLY WITH YOUR LEFT HAND. Rest a few moments then reverse the arm positions. Take a deep breath, expanding and raising your chest, then PRESS DOWN WITH YOUR LEFT FIST AGAINST UPWARD PRESSURE FROM YOUR RIGHT HAND.

Purpose
To strengthen, firm, tone and shape the muscles of the arms, concentrating on the triceps muscle at the rear of the upper arm. This three-headed muscle will contract strongly. It becomes flabby when not used sufficiently. It is worked in extending the arms from a bent position against resistance, as in pushing a weight overhead. During M6B its antagonist, the biceps, is exercised in the arm resisting pressure towards extension.

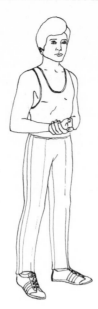

M7. The Cobra

Held Position

This lower back contraction exercise is taken from the ancient system of Hatha Yoga postures, whose practice is now popular in the West as a way to gain health and peace of mind in our present age of stress. Yoga postures were practised in India more than two thousand years ago. This posture has been named 'The Cobra' because the held position resembles that of a cobra rearing to strike.

Lie full length on the floor on your chest, stomach, pelvis, and legs. Keep your legs and your feet together. Place the palm of your right hand below your right shoulder and the palm of your left hand below your left shoulder and keep your elbows close to your body. The position resembles that adopted for starting the well-known 'push-up' exercise, but the Cobra Posture is more subtle in its execution and in its effects and does not require repetitions.

Breathe in, expanding your chest. Slowly raise your head and upper body using mainly the strength that comes from your lower back. Bend your back vertebra until your arms are straight. Your chest and upper abdomen will be raised off the floor, and your hands, your pelvis, your legs and your feet will be in contact with it. Tilt back your head and look diagonally upward. Release your breath evenly.

Contraction
SUSTAIN THE FINAL POSITION OF CONTRACTION OF THE LOWER BACK FOR THE REQUIRED NUMBER OF SECONDS. During the sustained contraction, take little breaths as required and stay perfectly still. Return *slowly* to the starting position of full length on the floor.

Purpose
The Cobra Posture stretches, strengthens, firms, tones and shapes the muscles of the back, arms, chest, and abdomen. The spine is limbered vertebra by vertebra from the lumber region to the neck, and the front of the body is beneficially stretched. The posture improves digestion, relieves constipation and promotes pelvic health.

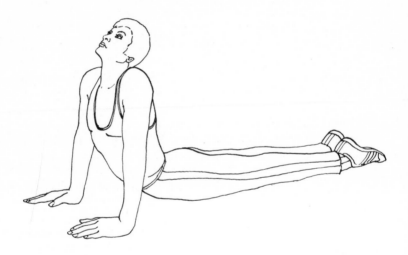

M8. The Curl Up

Held Position
Lie flat on your back, flex your legs and and draw your heels back towards your buttocks, keeping the soles of your feet flat on the floor. Interlock your fingers and hold your hands behind your neck. Breathe in, then exhaling, slowly raise your head, shoulders and upper back off the floor.

Contraction
HOLD THIS POSITION OF ABDOMINAL CONTRACTION FOR THE REQUIRED NUMBER OF SECONDS.

Drawing back your feet adds to the difficulty of starting to sit up. Additional resistance may be gained by holding a large book or other object behind your head or by resting your feet, with your legs fully extended, high up on a wall.

Purpose
This is almost entirely an abdominal exercise and you will be left in no doubt that the abdominal muscles are those most strongly contracted during the exercise. In an isotonic version of this exercise you would sit right up and perform a number of repetitions. In isometrics, you complete a partial sit up – a curl up – and then sustain the static contraction. Flab is removed from the middle region of the body and the abdominal wall is strengthened, firmed and toned.

An effective alternative version is to hook your toes under a heavy piece of furniture, your knees up and your abdomen close to your thighs with your hands behind your neck. Now lean back into the semi-sit-up position and hold the contraction. The farther you go back the greater the contraction. Abdominal trembling will set in as you reach your maximum point of endurance.

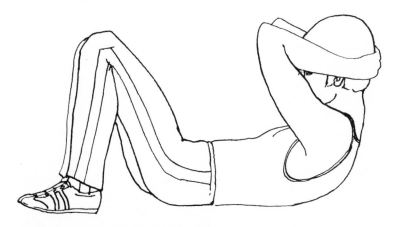

M9A. Abdominal Retraction

Held Position
Again we turn to yoga for a valuable and interesting exercise. Standing or sitting, you must exhale very fully. Exhale a little more after you feel your lungs are fully empty. Draw back the abdominal wall as far as it will go towards the spine, creating a large hollow. Actually, if you have exhaled thoroughly a

deep retraction should occur of its own accord, or almost of its own accord. This can be helped by rounding your back and leaning forward slightly from the waist. Observing the retraction in a mirror also helps.

Contraction

SUSTAIN THE RETRACTION OF THE ABDOMEN FOR FIVE OR SIX SECONDS. Rest a few moments then REPEAT THE RETRACTION. Hold your breath steady during the contraction, as letting the breath come back into the lungs would break the control.

Purpose

This is a superb muscle control for keeping the abdominal muscles and the internal organs they protect, in good condition. The internal organs are massaged and constipation is prevented. The supporting muscular 'corset' is strengthened, firmed, toned and shaped. Flab is removed.

The retraction may be repeated with advantage on other occasions during the day. Opportunities occur for unobtrusive practice in everyday life – the executive at his desk, the housewife before her stove, the motorist held up in a trafic jam.

M9B. Recti Isolation

A spectacular muscular display is possible after a really deep retraction on a full exhalation has been mastered. Lean forward a little and slightly round your back. Place the palm of your right hand on your right thigh and place the palm of your left hand on your left thigh. Exhale very fully and produce a deep abdominal retraction. BY MIND–MUSCLE CONTROL, ISOLATE AND BRING FORWARD THE TWO RECTUS MUSCLES IN THE CENTRE OF THE ABDOMEN. The recti appear as a thin wedge in the centre of the abdomen, from chest box to pubic bone, the retraction still showing to right and left of the isolated muscles. Experts can roll the abdominal muscles from side to side in a beneficial massaging action. Sustain the isolation of the recti for five or six seconds. Rest a few moments, then repeat the retraction and isolation.

Purpose

The benefits are as described for the Abdominal Retraction, but intensified.

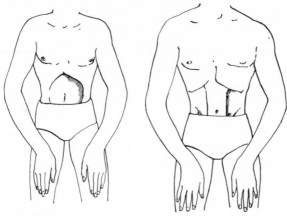

M10. Legs Raise

Held Position
Lie flat on your back with your legs fully extended together and your arms spread out diagonally on either side, the palms down on the floor. Take a deep breath, then raise your feet and legs to a height thirty to forty centimetres from the floor.

Contraction
HOLD THE LEGS IN THE RAISED POSITION FOR THE REQUIRED NUMBER OF SECONDS. Exhale slowly during the contraction and concentrate on the muscles of the lower abdomen. Lower your legs to the floor *slowly*.

Purpose
To strengthen the lower abdominal wall and to remove flab.

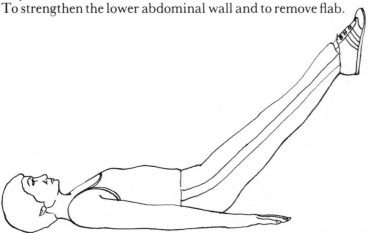

M11. Leg Press

Held Position
Here again a belt or a folded towel is used as an aid to
producing an isometric contraction. Lie flat on your back with
your legs extended together. Flex your right leg and bring
your right knee up and back until your upper leg is about
vertical and your upper and lower leg forms a right angle.
Loop the belt or the folded towel around the sole of your
raised right foot and draw it taut in such a way that your arms
are fully extended without raising your upper body and head
from the floor.

Contraction
Take a deep breath. TRY TO STRAIGHTEN YOUR
RIGHT LEG BUT PREVENT ANY MOVEMENT BY
PULLING BACK STRONGLY WITH YOUR ARMS. Rest
a few moments, then flex your left leg and loop the belt or
towel around the sole of your left foot and pull the belt or
towel taut as you did for contracting your right leg. Take a
deep breath. TRY TO STRAIGHTEN YOUR LEFT LEG
BUT PREVENT ANY MOVEMENT BY PULLING BACK
STRONGLY WITH YOUR ARMS. If the belt or towel has
been adjusted to the correct length, there should be no need to
raise your head or your back from the floor in countering the
thrust of each leg.

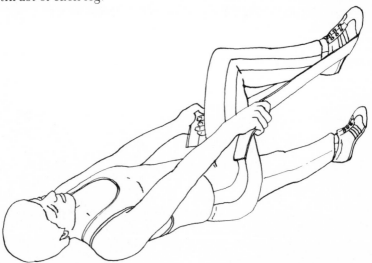

Purpose

To strengthen, firm, tone and shape the large group of muscles at the front of the upper leg (the extensors of the thigh). The hips also benefit. Trying to straighten a bent leg against resistance will always contract the frontal thigh muscles, which can be quite powerful. Their functioning – and that of their antagonist, the biceps of the thigh, at the rear of the upper leg – may be compared with that of the triceps and biceps of the upper arm. In each case, when one muscle is contracted either in flexion or in extension the antagonist muscle is relaxed and paying out slack.

M12. Toes and Feet Pointing

Held Position

Again use a belt or a folded towel. Sit on the floor with your legs extended together. Wrap the belt or the towel across your toes and the balls of your feet. Keep your legs straight. Pull the belt or the towel taut with your arms straight.

Contraction

Take a deep breath. CONCENTRATING ON YOUR TOES AND THE BALLS OF YOUR FEET, TRY TO PRESS THEM AWAY FROM YOU AND TO POINT YOUR TOES. PREVENT ANY MOVEMENT BY PULLING BACK HARD ON THE BELT OR TOWEL, LEANING BACK SLIGHTLY TO AID THIS.

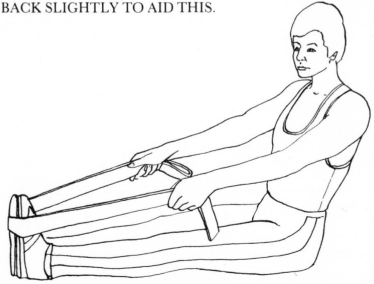

Purpose

This exercise will strengthen, firm, tone and shape the lower legs. You will be left in no doubt that the backs of the lower legs do most of the work in this exercise. Any position in which you try to point your toes against resistance will contract the calves.

SUMMARY OF PROGRAMME FOR MEN

To be consulted as a rapid reminder of the programme only after correct performance of each exercise, in every detail, has been memorized.

M1A. Brow Clasp

Clasp hands across brow. Press head forward and press hands back.

M1B. Head Clasp

Clasp hands across back of head. Press head back and press hands forward.

M1C. Head Turn

Palm of right hand against right temple. Block attempt to turn head to right. Repeat on left side of head.

M2 Bent Arms Press In

Hands together in front of chest. Press hands together.

M3. Bent Arms Pull Apart

Lock hands in front of chest. Try to pull them apart.

M4. Overhead Pull Out

Arms extended straight up, pulling belt or folded towel taut. Pull outwards.

M5A. Finger Strengthening

Spread fingers and thumbs and press them down on a table top.

M5B. Grip Strengthening
Squeeze a small hard ball or make tight fist first with one hand and then with the other hand.

M6A. Front Upper Arm Contraction
Flex right arm half-way at your side. Press left fist against right palm. Attempt to complete flexion of right arm. Repeat for left arm.

M6B. Rear Upper Arm Contraction
Flex right arm half-way at your side. Make fist of right hand. Place palm of left hand under right fist. Press down with right fist and press up with left hand. Repeat for left arm.

M7. The Cobra
Full length on floor face down. Hands below shoulders. Raise head and upper body to limit and sustain contraction.

M8. The Curl Up
Lie on back and draw back soles of feet. Clasp hands behind neck. Slowly raise head, shoulders and upper back and sustain contraction.

M9A. Abdominal Retraction
Exhale fully. Draw back abdominal wall. Sustain the retraction.

M9B. Recti Isolation
Breathe out and retract abdomen. Press central abdomen (recti) forward.

M10. Legs Raise
Lie on back legs extended together. Raise legs diagonally and sustain contraction.

M11. Leg Press
Lie on back. Flex right leg and loop a belt or folded towel around sole of raised foot. Pull taut. Attempt to straighten right leg but block by pulling back. Repeat for left leg.

M12. Toes and Feet Pointing
Sit on floor with legs extended together. Loop belt or towel across tops of feet. Try to point toes and feet but prevent by pulling back.

4.

Programme for Women

This programme will concentrate on helping those women who want to fashion a fit and shapely figure. At the same time strength and muscle tone will be increased and health will be enhanced.

Isometrics will trim your waistline, flatten your tummy muscles, round out your neck, slim your arms, taper your legs and raise and firm your bust. Of course it will not miraculously alter inherited bone structure and some associated bodily proportions, but the results, within reasonable expectations, can be highly satisfactory. Remoulding the figure to some extent toward more youthful and graceful lines is certainly not an exaggerated expectation.

Many women are suspicious of exercises that promote increased physical strength. They fear they will develop large muscles and a masculine appearance. This fear can be dismissed. In response to such exercise the female body retains its own nature. There are many examples of highly attractive women in sports and athletics.

Though gaining a more attractive and youthful appearance will be a frequent motive for women, there are also the important motives of attaining improved muscle tone and fitness, making life easier and more productive in numerous ways. The points made earlier about the value of having strength to cope with the demands of average activities and having more in reserve applies to women just as much as to men. You need strength to walk, to climb stairs, to do housework, to work in a garden, to drive a car, to work in an office, school or factory, to pick up and to hold a child – the last activity can be particularly fatiguing. It might further be mentioned that a strong fit body is a valuable preparation for the 'exercise' of giving birth.

Just standing up to the pressures of gravity for sixteen hours a day requires a certain level of strength. Without good muscular tone and healthy muscles the pressures of gravity result in a body that begins to droop and sag. Flesh on the chin, throat and breasts becomes loose and hangs; shoulders droop; the underarms become flabby; the stomach and the buttocks protrude and hang down. The whole upper body may press down concertina-like on to the hips. An overall system of body-firming and body-toning such as isometrics counters these effects of ageing. It is worth mentioning also that a strong body is less likely to suffer from minor aches and pains.

Instructions for Practice

General rules for practice were given in Chapter 2. The following points are worth noting again as they apply to the practice of the programme for women.

Breathing

Take a deep but *comfortable* breath before starting the contraction. Feel as though air is going down to your abdomen as well as expanding your chest. Breathe in and out through your nostrils unless they are blocked or the special nature of an exercise requires mouth breathing. Most women will find that if a deep breath is taken the air can be released slowly from the lungs during a contraction lasting eight to ten seconds. A quick breath may then be taken and released slowly until the contraction is completed. However, some women will find that the slow release of air following the first inhalation can continue comfortably for the maximum duration of a contraction, which is fifteen seconds. The important thing is to avoid discomfort or strain in your breathing. Take an extra breath if you really need it, but remember that unnecessary inhalations disrupt momentarily the steadiness of your pressure.

Force and Duration of Contraction

Category A (moderate strength requirements). Begin by sustaining each contraction for five seconds (a slow count of one, two, three, four, five). Add one second to the duration of each contraction at the end of each week until the duration of each contraction is ten seconds. Exert strong pressure without straining: about three-quarters of your maximum strength.

Category B (standard strength requirements). Begin by sustaining each contraction for six seconds (a slow count of one, two, three, four, five, six). Add one second per week until the duration of each contraction is twelve seconds. Exert powerful pressure, that is about ninety per cent of your maximum strength.

Category C (maximum strength requirements). Begin by sustaining each contraction for nine seconds. Add one second per week until the duration of each contraction is fifteen seconds. Exert maximum pressure.

All categories. To avoid muscle strain, do not start with a sudden jerk. Apply steady pressure.

Women desiring strength for sports and athletics should practise the programme for women for six to eight weeks to condition their muscles to static contractions and then move on to the programme for muscular power.

W1A. Brow Clasp

Held Position
Stand up straight, your head and your back poised in line. In keeping the back straight there should be ease not rigidity. Spread your feet a little apart to give firm support to your upright posture. Interlace your fingers, raise your elbows out full width to either side and press the palms of your hands horizontally across your forehead. (See M1A for illustration.)

Contraction
Take a deep breath. PRESS YOUR HEAD FORWARD AND AT THE SAME TIME PULL BACKWARD WITH YOUR CLASPED HANDS. Your head should not move during the contraction.

Purpose
To round out the front of the neck. Poor tone in this area is one of the first signs of departing youthfulness. The front of the neck is exercised by pressing your head forward against resistance. The arms and shoulders also benefit from this isometric contraction.

W1B. Head Clasp

Held Position
Again stand easily erect. Again interlock your fingers and hold your elbows out wide to either side. But this time turn the palms of your hands forward and carry your hands over your

head and press your palms horizontally across the base of your skull.

Contraction
Take a deep breath, then PRESS BACKWARD WITH YOUR HEAD AND AT THE SAME TIME PRESS FORWARD WITH YOUR CLASPED HANDS. The result should be a contraction of your neck muscles but no movement of your head

Purpose
This exercise will round out, strengthen, firm and tone the muscles at the back of the neck. There is also some exercise for the arms and shoulders.

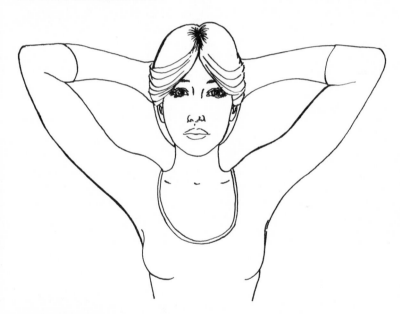

W1C. Head Turn

Held Position
Stand easily erect with your feet a little apart and with your head and your back in poised line. Look straight ahead without staring. Place the palm of your right hand horizontally across your right temple just above your right ear so that your fingers point toward the back of your head. Hold your right elbow out wide to your right side. (See M1C for illustration.)

Contraction
Take a deep breath, then TRY TO TURN YOUR HEAD
TO YOUR RIGHT BUT AT THE SAME TIME PRESS IN
WITH YOUR RIGHT HAND SO THAT THERE IS A
CONTRACTION OF YOUR NECK MUSCLES
WITHOUT ANY MOVEMENT OF YOUR HEAD. Rest a
few moments, then REPEAT TO THE LEFT SIDE,
PRESSING YOUR HEAD TO THE LEFT AND
RESISTING WITH YOUR LEFT ARM. The palm of your
left hand is pressed horizontally above your left ear.

Purpose
This will strengthen, firm, tone and shape the muscles at the
sides of the neck. The chief muscle worked is the sterno
mastoid. The right side of the neck contracts on blocking an
attempt to turn your head to the right and the left side of the
neck contracts on blocking an attempt to turn your head to your
left.

W2A. Press In At Bust Level

Held Position
Stand upright, your feet a little apart for stability, with your
chest about ten centimetres from the edge of an open door.
Bend your arms and place the palms of your hands before
your chest on either side of the door edge, with your fingers
pointing upward. Lift your elbows out wide to either side until
your forearms are parallel to the floor and your upper and
lower arms form right angles.

Contraction
Take a deep breath, expanding and raising your chest, then
PRESS YOUR HANDS IN STRONGLY AS THOUGH TO
BRING YOUR PALMS TOGETHER.

Purpose
This will strengthen, firm, tone and shape the chest muscles
(the pectorals) underlying your bust. The effect is to support
and raise the bust and to improve your appearance. The
firming, supporting and raising effect will soon be
experienced.

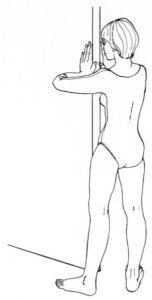

W2B. Bent Arms Press In Overhead

Held Position
The Press In on the door described in W2A could also be performed by pressing the palms of your hands together in front of your chest as described and illustrated in the programme for men M2. We will employ the 'hands together' method now to produce a high chest contraction. Hold the palms of your hands together in front of you, your upper and lower arms forming right angles. Raise your hands to a position directly above your head. Keep your elbows out to either side and level with your ears.

Contraction
Take a deep breath, expanding and raising your chest, then PRESS YOUR HANDS TOGETHER STRONGLY. Stand easily upright, your feet slightly apart, looking straight ahead as you perform the contraction, which should produce no movement in your arms, body or legs.

Purpose
For a high firm bust. The pectorals which underlie and support the breasts are exercised in W2B in their top fibres. The arms and shoulders are at the same time firmed and toned.

Several variations of these Press Ins are possible. You may press in on a door in a similar manner to that described in W2A but standing further back from the edge of the door and extending your arms to full length, or take an in between position with the palms of your hands on either side of the door with your fingers pointing away from you and your elbows kept in against your sides. These variations will contract the chest muscles which support the breasts at slightly different angles to those experienced in exercises W2A and W2B.

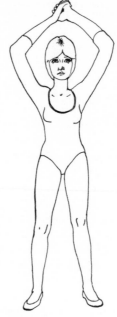

W3A. Finger Strengthening
It may be thought that strong hands are not as essential for women as they are for men. In fact, a few seconds regular exercise for your fingers and your grip will help you ward off weakness in the hands and in the forearms as age advances.

To strengthen the fingers, stretch and spread them then PRESS YOUR FINGERS DOWN ON A TABLE TOP OR ANY OTHER UNYIELDING SURFACE.

W3B. Grip Strengthening
To strengthen your grip and your forearms, SQUEEZE YOUR FISTS VERY TIGHTLY or SQUEEZE HARD ON A SMALL HARD BALL, FIRST WITH ONE HAND AND THEN WITH THE OTHER HAND.

Purpose
To strengthen and retain strength in your fingers, your grip, your wrists and your forearms.

W4. Doorway Press Out

Held Position
Stand in the centre of the frame of a doorway. Stand easily erect and spread your feet comfortably apart to provide a solid base. Now clench your fists and press the sides of your fists against either side of the door frame, about level with the top of your head. This means that your arms will be slightly flexed.

Contraction
Breathe in deeply, expanding your chest and back, then PRESS OUT AGAINST THE DOOR JAMBS. Your body should not move during the contraction and you should avoid thrusting your head forward.

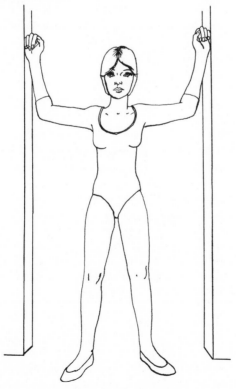

Purpose

To strengthen, firm, tone and shape the muscles at the rear of the upper arm (the triceps) which are responsible for extending the arm. These muscles become loose and flabby in many women, due to inadequate exercise of them. The biceps at the front of the upper arm, which is responsible for flexing the arm, is exercised in the preceding Press Ins W2A and W2B.

W5. Abdominal Retraction

Held Position

This is a yoga exercise for abdominal health. Standing or sitting, you exhale very fully. A useful tip is to exhale a little more after you already feel you have emptied your lungs of air. Draw back your abdominal wall between chest and pelvis. If your exhalation has been complete the retraction will be effortless or nearly effortless. A deep retraction is aided by rounding your back slightly and leaning forward slightly from your waist. Observing this muscle control in a mirror will be found helpful in early practice. The nature of this exercise is a muscle control and good mind-muscle rapport develops quickly. (See M9A for illustration.)

Contraction

SUSTAIN THE DEEP ABDOMINAL RETRACTION FOR FIVE OR SIX SECONDS. The breath has to be held in check during the contraction; if air enters the lungs the retraction will collapse. Release the abdominal retraction and breathe normally for a few moments. Then exhale fully again and REPEAT HOLDING IN THE ABDOMINAL WALL FOR FIVE OR SIX SECONDS.

Purpose

This exercise will take flab from the abdomen and strengthen, firm and tone it. The retraction will also massage the internal abdominal organs and promote easy natural elimination of food waste material from the colon.

W6. The Bow

Held Position

This is another yoga posture. It takes its name from the appearance of the held position. The spine, trunk and legs take the shape of a bow and the arms hold the ankles and are pulled taut like a bow string.

Lie flat on your abdomen with your knees a little apart. Flex your legs and bring your heels up and back towards your buttocks. Reach back and grasp your right ankle with your right hand and grasp your left ankle with your left hand, with your thumbs alongside your fingers. This means lifting your head and your chest off the floor. Your back is arched into a bow shape.

Contraction

Breathe in, then LIFT YOUR HEAD, YOUR NECK AND YOUR SHOULDERS AS HIGH AS YOU CAN WHILE AT THE SAME TIME, PULLING STRONGLY ON YOUR ANKLES WITH YOUR ARMS. The effect is to intensify the bow shape of the body. Some extremely supple Yogins can actually place the soles of their feet on top of their heads. Hold the Bow Posture steadily for the required number of seconds. Spreading your legs apart makes this exercise easier and may be essential in early practice. Later you should be able to gradually bring your legs closer together until finally you can sustain the 'bow' with your legs touching together along their full length.

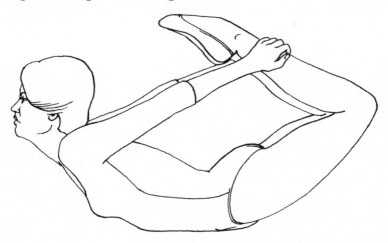

Purpose
This will stretch, strengthen, firm, tone and shape the muscles of your back, thighs, abdomen, chest, arms, shoulders and neck. Your spine, your hip joints and your shoulder joints are limbered. Your back muscles are strengthened. The front of your body – including your legs, abdomen, chest, arms, throat and jawline – is stretched, firmed and toned. Your stomach muscles are massaged and your abdominal organs are stimulated and toned.

W7. Buttock Firming

Held Position .
Stand up straight with your hands on your hips and your feet spread comfortably apart.

Contraction
Breathe in. Through mind-muscle control DRAW IN AND CONTRACT THE BUTTOCK MUSCLES FIRMLY. You will assist the contraction if you pull your feet back and in against the resistance of the floor on which you stand, though without actually moving your feet. Rest a few moments then REPEAT THE CONTRACTION OF THE BUTTOCKS.

Purpose
To firm the buttocks. If you squeeze in the gripping muscles of the vagina at the same time that you contract the buttocks you will add the benefit of promoting sexual health and fitness. This is an exercise taught in the old love manuals of the East.

W8. Legs Squeeze In

Held Position
For a Legs Squeeze In you should find an object thirty to forty centimetres wide. Possible objects are the legs of a table chair, a hassock, a pouffe, a wastepaper basket or container, or a bucket. Sit on the floor with your legs extended fully. Help your balance by placing your right hand on the floor behind your right hip and by placing your left hand on the floor behind your left hip. Keep your arms straight. Place your feet on either side of the object. Grip the object firmly with your feet, keeping your legs and heels in contact with the floor.

Contraction
Take a deep breath and SQUEEZE IN HARD WITH
YOUR FEET AS THOUGH TRYING TO CRUSH THE
OBJECT AND BRING YOUR FEET TOGETHER.

Purpose
To strengthen, firm, tone and shape the muscles of the inner
thighs which bring the legs together. Fat is removed from the
legs and the hips also benefit.

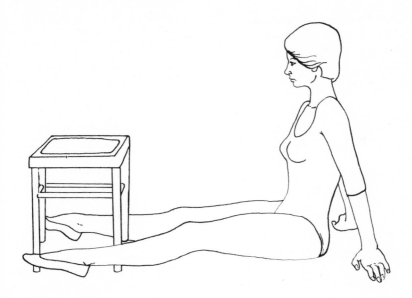

W9. Legs Pull Apart

Held Position
This is the converse of the Legs Squeeze In described in the
preceding contraction W8 and exercises other parts of the
legs. No object is required this time, as the strength of one leg
is pitted against the power of the other but the legs are locked
together at the ankles.

Retain the sitting on floor position of exercise W8, having
pushed away the chair, or whatever object was used to block
the bringing together of the legs. Support your balance as
before by placing your arms behind either hip. Cross your feet
at your ankles, your left foot on top of the right or your right
foot on top of left, and lock your legs firmly together.

Contraction
Breathe in, keep your legs straight and your feet and ankles firmly crossed, then TRY TO FORCE YOUR LEGS APART. Block any movement.

Purpose
In attempting to pull your legs apart against resistance the outside muscles of the thighs are contracted. This and the preceding exercise thus help to streamline and round out the legs.

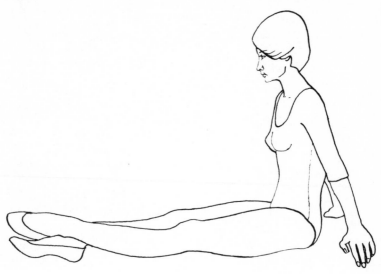

W10. Lower Leg Contractions

Held Position
This is a double exercise which contracts first the fronts of the lower legs and then the calf muscles at the backs of the lower legs.

Sit on the floor, your legs fully extended, assisting your balance with straight arms as in the two preceding exercises W8 and W9. No object is required. Keep your legs together.

Contractions
Breathe in then DRAW YOUR TOES AND FEET UP AND BACK TOWARDS YOUR KNEES. Your heels should stay in contact with the floor. Only your feet should move. Sustain the contraction for the required number of seconds.

Rest a few moments. NOW POINT YOUR TOES AND FEET FORWARD AND AWAY FROM YOU. Your legs should remain fully extended and only your feet should move. Sustain the contraction for the required number of seconds.

Purpose
Raising the foot against the ankle joint contracts the tibialis anticus at the front of the lower leg. Pointing the toes and foot away from you contracts the calf muscle at the rear of the lower leg. The intensity of the contraction may be increased later by holding a belt or a folded towel taut around the tops of the feet as described and illustrated in the final exercise of the programme for men M12.

SUMMARY OF
PROGRAMME FOR WOMEN

To be consulted as a rapid reminder of the programme only after correct performance of each exercise, in every detail, has been memorized.

W1A. Brow Clasp
Clasp hands across brow. Press head forward and press hands back.

W1B. Head Clasp
Clasp hands across back of head. Press head back and press hands forward.

W1C. Head Turn
Palm of right hand against right temple. Block attempt to turn head to right. Repeat on left side of head.

W2A. Press In At Bust Level
Squeeze in on edge of door, elbows held wide.

W2B. Bent Arms Press In Overhead
Arms bent, press hands together over head.

W3A. Finger Strengthening

Spread fingers and thumbs and press them down on a table top.

W3B. Grip Strengthening

Squeeze a small hard ball or make a tight fist first with one hand and then with the other hand.

W4. Doorway Press Out

Stand in doorway and press sides of fists against jambs.

W5. Abdominal Retraction

Exhale fully. Draw back abdominal wall. Sustain the retraction.

W6. The Bow

Face down, grasp ankles and pull body and arms into bow shape. Sustain the bow posture.

W7. Buttock Firming

Stand upright and contract buttocks through mind-muscle control.

W8. Legs Squeeze in

Sit on floor with legs extended. Squeeze feet in on object.

W9. Legs Pull Apart

Sit on floor and cross feet at ankles. Try to pull legs apart.

W10. Lower Leg Contractions

Sit on floor with legs extended. Draw feet back towards your knees. Point toes and feet forward.

5.

Programme for Muscle Power

Athletes, body-builders, sportsmen and sportswomen require muscular power for their particular interests. The programme for men given earlier is already geared to exercising the main muscle masses, but general strength requirements are taken into account. The following programme aims directly for great muscle power in the strongest areas of the body. Apply almost maximum pressure. Perform each contraction twice (except for the P1 neck contractions).

Athletes, sportsmen and sportswomen will be familiar with those muscles and muscle groups important to their sport or athletic event. Footballers, jumpers and sprinters will wish to pay particular attention to strengthening their legs. Swimmers will want powerful shoulders, throwers in field events will seek powerful arms and shoulders. Up to five additional contractions may be added to your programme to cater for special strength needs. However, it should not be forgotten that strength comes from the whole body and that the main muscle masses of the body should always be at the centre of the isometrics programme.

It is also worth trying to find held positions for static contractions that simulate athletic or sporting performance. These positions will be known to each reader. For example, a sprinter could take up the starting position for a race but use his or her arms to block a start and produce a static contraction in the muscles of the legs which produce the thrust that takes the sprinter explosively out of the starting blocks. Best results are obtained if the action of the athlete or sportsman or sportswoman is posed statically at three points – near the start of the action, about the middle, and near the end. In the example already given of the sprinter, static contractions should be produced shortly after the legs begin to straighten, at mid-point, and finally near to straightening. Similarly, say, for a shot-putter. A door jamb, wall edge, or metal bar could provide the unyielding resistance. Static contractions in the important muscles should be produced at a point shortly after the shot leaves the cradle of the neck, at about a half-way extension of the driving arm, and finally with the arm coming close to extension. You should have little difficulty in working out held positions to contract muscles most conducive to greater success in your sport or athletic event.

Instructions for Practice
General rules for practice were given in Chapter 2. The following points are worth noting again as they apply to practice of the programme for muscle power.

Breathing
Take a deep but *comfortable* breath before starting the contraction. Feel as though air is going down to your abdomen as well as expanding your chest. Breathe in and out through your nostrils unless they are blocked or the special nature of an exercise requires mouth breathing. Most people will find that if a deep breath is taken the air can be released slowly from the lungs during a contraction lasing eight to ten seconds. A quick breath may then be taken and released slowly until the contraction is completed. Some people will experience no difficulty in exhaling during the whole of a contraction lasting fifteen seconds. The important thing is to avoid discomfort or strain in your breathing. Take an extra breath if you really need it, but remember that unnecessary inhalations disrupt momentarily the steadiness of your pressure.

Force and Duration of Contraction
This is not a programme for Category A people – those with moderate strength requirements. Some people may wish to build considerable muscle power without having the aims of an athlete and for them Category B instructions are given. If your sights are on the maximum build up of strength then your contractions should be of the duration and strength given under the instructions for Category C.

Category B (standard strength requirements). Begin by

sustaining each contraction for six seconds (a slow count of one, two, three, four, five six). Add one second per week until the duration of each contraction is twelve seconds. Exert powerful pressure that is *almost* maximum strength.

Category C (maximum strength requirements). Begin by sustaining each contraction for nine seconds. Add one second per week until the duration of each contraction is fifteen seconds. Exert maximum pressure.

All categories. To avoid muscle strain, do not start with a sudden jerk. Apply steady pressure.

Neck Contractions

The contractions for the muscles at the front, back and sides of the neck as given in the Programme for Men M1A, M1B and M1C should be performed. This means pressing your head forward against resistance, backward against resistance and to each side against resistance respectively. In the earlier programme your hands and arms provided the resistance and may do so again, but the power seeker may prefer to use either of two alternatives. The first is use of a belt – a webbed belt is excellent – or a folded towel to wrap across the brow to exercise the muscles at the front of the neck and across the base of the skull to contract the muscles at the back of the neck. Placing a hand across the temple for attempts at turning your head to the sides is still the best way to provide resistance for the muscles at the sides of the neck.

The second alternative to using the hands to block attempted movement of the head is to press your forehead, back of head or side of head against a doorway, placing a folded towel or other pad between your head and the door jamb for protection. This is a formidable method that may appeal to persons seeking a powerful neck. The methods can now be looked at in more detail.

P1A. Head Forward Press

Held Position
Stand upright close to the door jamb. Place your forehead against the frame of the door, with a pad between your head and the wood. Take a deep breath then PRESS FORWARD STRONGLY WITH YOUR HEAD. At the same time grip the door jamb with both hands. The muscles at the front of your neck will contract.

P1B. Head Backward Press

Held Position
Stand up straight with your back close to a door jamb. Place the back of your head against the frame of the door, with a pad protecting your skull. Take a deep breath then PRESS BACKWARD STRONGLY WITH YOUR HEAD. At the same time grip the door jamb with both hands. The muscles at the back of the neck are contracted.

P1C. Head Sideward Press

Held Position
Stand erect in a doorway so that the right side of your chest, hip and legs are against a door jamb. Your right shoulder and right arm should be pulled back to fit in against the outside wood of the door frame, your right arm fully extended and your right hand gripping the wood. Place the right side of your head against the jamb, with a pad between your head and the wood.

Contraction
Take a deep breath then PRESS THE RIGHT SIDE OF YOUR HEAD STRONGLY AGAINST THE DOOR JAMB. The muscles at the right side of your neck will contract. Turn round and repeat the neck contraction PRESSING THE LEFT SIDE OF YOUR HEAD STRONGLY AGAINST THE DOOR JAMB. The muscles at the left side of your neck will contract.

In this power-packing programme I suggest two further exercises for the neck muscles, in which resistance blocks attempted movements from two different held positions.

P1D. Head Lowering

Held Position
Stand comfortably erect. Raise your chin and tilt your head back. Cup your chin in the palm of your right hand (left hand if you are left-handed) with your upper arm in against your chest. Keep your mouth closed and your tongue flat at the bottom of your mouth with the tip of your tongue behind your lower teeth. Breathe through your nostrils.

Contraction
Inhale through your nostrils then TRY TO LOWER YOUR CHIN BUT BLOCK ANY MOVEMENT OF YOUR HEAD BY PRESSING UP ON YOUR CHIN WITH THE HEEL OF YOUR RIGHT HAND.

Chief Muscles Exercised
These are the muscles at the front and the sides of the neck responsible for lowering your head and also your jaw muscles.

P1E. Head Raising

Held Position
Here again the title of the exercise refers to the direction of an *attempted* movement and not to the movement itself. Stand upright, your head and your back in poised line. Lower your chin towards your chest. Interlace your fingers and clasp the palms of your hands across the crown of your head, holding your elbows out wide to either side.

Contraction
Take a deep breath then TRY TO RAISE YOUR HEAD UP AND BACK TO A LEVEL POSITION, BUT PREVENT ANY MOVEMENT OF THE HEAD BY PRESSING DOWN WITH YOUR HANDS.

Chief Muscles Exercised
These are muscles at the back of your neck responsible for lifting your head. Also your arms and shoulders to some extent.

P2. Chair Shrug

Held Position
This seated exercise packs power into the shoulders and into the upper back. Your own weight on a chair provides the unyielding resistance. Sit up straight on a table chair. Grip the right side of the seat of the chair with your right hand and grip the left side of the seat with your left hand. Grip firmly. Your body should be in a straight line from hips to head, and your arms should be fully extended. If you find that your arms are not straight, place a cushion, cushions or other object on the chair seat to bring you up to the required height. Your feet should be flat on the floor and your knees a little apart.

Contraction

Take a deep breath, expanding your chest and back, then
TRY TO SHRUG YOUR SHOULDERS. Because your fully
extended arms are gripping firmly the seat of the chair you
will not be able to raise your shoulders, but once again it is the
attempt that produces a static contraction. Rest a minute or so
and then repeat the contraction.

Chief Muscles Exercised

These are the shoulders and the trapezius which runs across
the upper back. The contraction of the trapezius will show at
both sides of the neck if you gaze at your reflection in a mirror
as you perform this exercise. This muscle acts as a brace for
the shoulders and if it becomes weak and loses tone the
shoulders will droop. It raises, lowers, and rotates the
shoulder-blades.

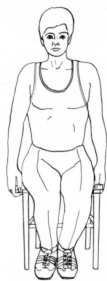

P3A. Wall Push

Held Position

The principle behind isometric contraction exercises should
already be perfectly clear to you: a static contraction
produced by attempts at movement being blocked by an
unyielding resistance. A solid wall provides unyielding
resistance for the seeker of muscular power.

For a frontal 'assault' on the wall, place the palms of your
hands flat on the wall at shoulder height and at shoulders'

width. Lean slightly forward from the waist to push with straight arms. Place your left leg in advance of the right leg; bend the left leg slightly but keep the right leg straight.

Contraction
Take a deep breath, expanding your chest, then PUSH POWERFULLY AGAINST THE WALL WITH YOUR EXTENDED ARMS, as though trying to push down the wall. If you have selected a solid wall you are unlikely to cause any damage, but team efforts should be discouraged unless you are demolishing a building. The USA weight-lifting team took to isometrics with such enthusiasm that they pushed down a hotel wall in Kiev. Rest a few moments, then take a deep breath and PUSH POWERFULLY AGAINST THE WALL WITH YOUR EXTENDED ARMS, BUT THIS TIME HAVE YOUR SLIGHTLY FLEXED RIGHT LEG IN FRONT OF YOUR FULLY EXTENDED LEFT LEG.

Chief Muscles Exercised
All the main muscle masses of your body are involved: those of your arms, your chest, your back, your abdomen and your legs.

P3B. Two Arms Push Back

Held Position
Stand easily upright thirty to forty centimetres from a wall. Your head and your back should be in a poised straight line. Spread your feet apart a little to provide a good base for muscular effort. Keep your head level and look straight ahead. Hold your arms straight down by your sides, the palms of your hands facing back towards the wall. Reach straight back with both hands and place your palms flat against the wall. The distance between your hands will be that between your shoulders.

Contraction
Breathe in, expanding and raising your chest, then PRESS BACK HARD WITH THE PALMS OF YOUR HANDS AGAINST THE WALL. Retain your upright posture during the contraction. Continue to look straight ahead. Grip the floor firmly with your feet to prevent any body movement. Rest about a minute and then repeat the contraction.

Chief Muscles Exercised

This Two Arms Push Back against a wall will strengthen the muscles of your rear upper arm (the triceps), your shoulders, and your upper back.

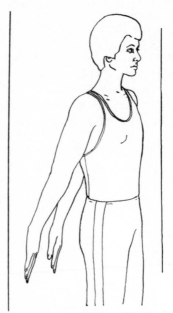

P4. Two Hands Press Overhead

Held Position

This isometric exercise simulates the first of the three lifts which decide Olympic and world weight-lifting championships. In the Two Hands Press, the bar of the bar-bell is gripped at shoulders' width and pulled up onto the chest. The lifter has to keep his back and his legs straight as he 'presses' the bar-bell to full arms length overhead. It requires concentrated power in the arms and in the upper body. There must be no jerk from the knees.

For the blocked isometric version an unyielding overhead object must be found, at the right height for you to stand erect, with your feet comfortably apart and your arms bent as though the two hands press described above has been 'frozen' part way in its execution. The most effective position is just over half-way through an imaginary arm extension against resistance. A doorway will serve for most people, though the shorter person may need to look for a low doorway or provide some safe platform to stand on.

Contraction
Take a deep breath, expanding and raising your chest, then THRUST UP POWERFULLY WITH BOTH ARMS AS THOUGH ATTEMPTING TO STRAIGHTEN YOUR ARMS. Keep your back upright and your legs straight. Rest about a minute and then repeat the contraction.

Chief Muscles Exercised
These are your rear upper arms, your shoulders and your upper back.

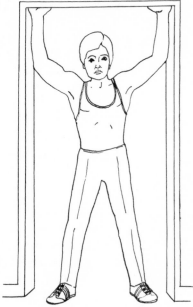

P5. Press Out In Doorway

Held Position
Again stand in the middle of a doorway, with your legs spread comfortably apart. This time bend your arms and place the palm of your right hand against the door-post to your right and place the palm of your left hand against the door-post to your left. Your upright fingers should be a little above shoulders' height.

Contraction
Breathe in, expanding and raising your chest, then PRESS OUT POWERFULLY as though trying to widen the doorway. Rest about a minute then repeat the press out.

Chief Muscles Exercised

Your wrists, forearms, rear upper arms, shoulders and upper back are exercised with this contraction.

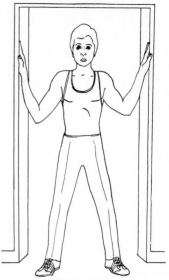

P6A. Table Press Up

These two contractions, P6A and P6B, are for the muscles of the front upper arm and the rear upper arm respectively. They pack power into the arms for both flexing and extending them against resistance. Versions of the two exercises have already been described in the programme for men, exercises M6A and M6B. Then the strength of one arm was pitted against the strength of the other arm to produce static contractions. Here, we utilize a heavy table.

Held Position

Sit up straight about thirty centimetres from a heavy table, your head and back in line. Keeping your upper arms in against your sides, bend your arms and place the palms of your hands under the table top. Sit on a chair of the right height to produce right angles between your upper and lower arms in the held position, or very close to it. The distance between your two hands should be the same as that between your shoulders.

Contraction

Keep your back erect and look straight ahead. Take a deep breath, expanding your chest, then PRESS UP STRONGLY

WITH YOUR HANDS without moving your arms or any part of your body. The table should provide an immovable resistance. Rest about a minute then repeat the press up.

Chief Muscles Exercised
The muscles at the front of the upper arm, the biceps brachialis, are responsible for flexing it. A 'coconut' development of the biceps muscle had long been associated with manly strength. Note that as the front of the upper arm contracts the rear of the upper arm relaxes. The biceps brachialis is used in lifting weights from below, in digging, shovelling, climbing, and so on.

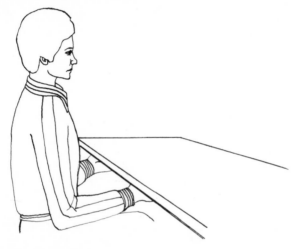

P6B. Table Press Down

Held Position
Sit up straight about thirty centimetres from a heavy table, your head and back in line, as for the Table Press Up contraction P6A. This time instead of placing the palms of your hands below the table top place them *on top* at shoulders' width. Keep your elbows and your upper arms in against your body. The whole of each hand should be flat on the surface of the table top and you should sit at a height which allows for an angle of ninety degrees between the upper and lower sections of each arm.

Contraction
Take a deep breath, expanding your chest and back. Keeping your back erect and looking straight ahead, PRESS DOWN

HARD WITH YOUR HANDS ON THE TABLE TOP.
Rest about a minute then repeat the press down.

Chief Muscles Exercised
Mainly the triceps, a three-headed muscle at the rear of the
upper arm which is responsible for straightening the elbow. It
is the antagonist muscle of the biceps, which you contracted in
performing P6A, contracting when the biceps is relaxed and
relaxing and paying out slack when the biceps contracts. The
triceps is used in throwing, bowling, punching, pushing and
overhead lifting.

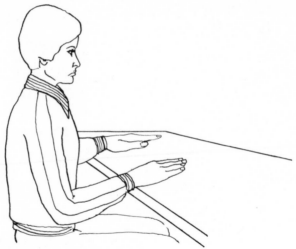

P7. Extended Arms Press Down

Held Position
This contraction has similarities to the preceding contraction
P6B for the rear upper arm, but the back muscles are strongly
contracted by sitting well back from a table, extending your
arms to full length and placing the palms of your hands flat on
the table top at shoulders' width. Place the whole of each hand
on the table top and sit up straight looking directly ahead.

Contraction
Take a deep breath, expanding your chest and back, then
PRESS DOWN STRONGLY ON THE TABLE (OR
DESK) TOP WITH BOTH HANDS. Your arms should stay
fully extended during the contraction and your head and back
should stay in a poised vertical line without moving. Rest
about a minute then press down again.

The exercise may also be performed using one arm at a time, sitting sideways to the table or desk. Again sit up straight and press down strongly with first the extended right arm and then the left arm.

Chief Muscles Exercised
These are the broad powerful latissimus dorsi of the upper back and flanks. In pressing down your arm against resistance this muscle shows in relief curving around the shoulder blade (scapula). It operates strongly in pulling the arms down and back against resistance, in chinning the bar, in rowing, in climbing, and so on.

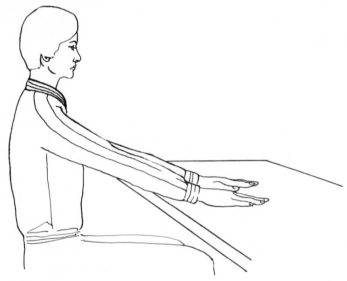

P8. Straight Arms Pull Over

Held Position
Lie full length on your back and extend your arms fully behind your head. Your legs should also be fully extended, but relaxed. The spacing of your hands should be about the same width as your shoulders. Place the palms of your hands beneath the seat of a chair that is about forty centimetres above the floor. It may be necessary to place a weight on the chair to keep it from moving during the contraction.

Contraction
Breathe in, expanding your chest. Keeping your arms straight and your back flat on the floor, TRY TO RAISE YOUR

HANDS AS THOUGH TO BRING YOUR ARMS UP TO A VERTICAL POSITION. Rest about a minute then repeat the contraction.

Chief Muscles Exercised
The Straight Arms Pull Over – imaged but not accomplished – strengthens, shapes and develops the muscles of your chest and back, and stretches and mobilizes the thorax thus aiding breathing and circulation.

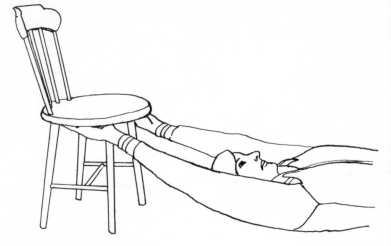

P9. Advanced Curl Up

Held Position
This is a more advanced version of the partial sit up described in the programme for men M8. Resistance is increased by extending your legs together high up on a wall. Clasp your hands behind your neck.

Contraction
Breathe in, then exhaling, slowly raise your head, shoulders and upper back off the floor. HOLD THE PARTIAL SIT UP FOR THE REQUIRED NUMBER OF SECONDS. Slowly lower your head and upper body to the floor. Rest about a minute then repeat the contraction.

Chief Muscles Exercised
This exercise will strongly contract the abdominal wall, the muscular 'corset' four layers thick between the diaphragm and the pelvis.

P10. Legs Thrust

Held Position
As for the Two Hands Press Overhead, P4, you stand in the middle of a doorway and press the palms of your hands up against the frame at the same width as your shoulders. As most of the work has to be done by the legs, you reverse the roles of the arms and legs that were taken in the press ups. You keep your arms straight throughout the contraction, but bend your legs, which should be spread comfortably apart for stability.

Contraction
Take a deep breath, expanding your chest, then THRUST UP WITH YOUR LEGS, ATTEMPTING TO STRAIGHTEN THEM, BUT FAILING BECAUSE YOUR STRAIGHT ARMS AND STRAIGHT BACK BLOCKS THE EFFORT OF YOUR LEGS. Rest about a minute then repeat the legs thrust.

Chief Muscles Exercised
The extensors of the thighs, the large frontal thigh muscles that straighten the legs against resistance. Power in these muscles is essential for most sports and for athletics. They are worked to great effect in running, jumping, rowing, climbing, kicking a ball, dancing, weight-lifting, putting the shot, and so on.

P11. Side Foot Raise Against Wall

Held Position
Stand easily erect with a wall thirty to forty centimetres to your right side. Keeping upright, raise your right foot out to the side and hold the side of your foot against the wall.

Contraction
Take a deep breath, then PRESS YOUR RAISED FOOT AGAINST THE WALL. Keep your leg straight and keep as steady and erect as you can manage. Rest a few moments and then turn round and repeat, PRESSING AGAINST THE WALL WITH YOUR LEFT FOOT. Contract each leg again.

Chief Muscles Exercised

This contraction exercises the muscles at the outside of your thighs and your hips. These muscles, which raise your legs sideways, are often under-exercised. This exercise will add to the general strength of the legs.

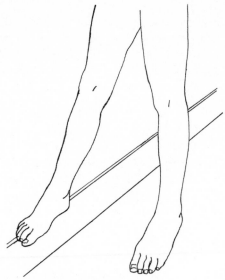

P12. Heel Raise Against Wall

Held Position

Stand upright with your back thirty to forty centimetres from a wall. Bend your right leg and raise your right heel slowly backward until your heel rests against the wall.

Contraction

Take a deep breath, expanding and raising your chest, then TRY HARD TO RAISE YOUR RIGHT HEEL FURTHER. Keep standing upright. Rest a few moments, then repeat with your left leg. PRESS YOUR LEFT HEEL BACK HARD AGAINST THE WALL. Contract each leg again.

Chief Muscles Exercised

The biceps of the thigh at the rear of the upper leg will contract. It flexes your leg just as the biceps of the arm flexes your arm. This muscle is usually under-exercised in everyday living and by strengthening it you will add to the overall strength of your legs.

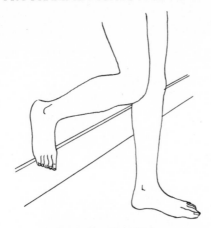

SUMMARY OF PROGRAMME FOR MUSCLE POWER

To be consulted as a rapid reminder of the programme only after correct performance of each exercise has been memorized in every detail.

P1A. Head Forward Press
Forehead against door jamb. Press head forward.

P1B. Head Backward Press
Back of head against door jamb. Press head backward.

P1C. Head Sideward Press
Side of head against door jamb. Press head to side. Turn round and repeat with other side of head.

P1D. Head Lowering
Tilt head back and cup chin in palm of one hand. Try to lower chin but block with hand.

P1E. Head Raising
Lower chin towards chest. Clasp hands across crown of head. Try to raise head but block with hands.

P2. Chair Shrug
Sit upright and grip chair seat. Try to shrug shoulders.

P3A. Wall Push
Palms of hands on wall at shoulders' width. Attempt to push down wall.

P3B. Two Arms Push Back
Stand back to wall. Reach back and press palms against wall.

P4. Two Hands Press Overhead
Stand in doorway, palms overhead on door frame with arms bent. Attempt to straighten arms.

P5. Press Out in Doorway
Stand in doorway. Palms against jambs. Press out as though trying to widen doorway.

P6A. Table Press Up
Sit with hands under a table. Press hands up.

P6B. Table Press Down
Sit with hands on table top. Press hands down.

P7. Extended Arms Press Down
Sit with extended arms on table top. Press hands down.

P8. Straight Arms Pull Over
Lying on back, arms extended behind head and palms under chair seat. Try to raise hands.

P9. Advanced Curl Up
Lie on back, legs together, feet high on wall. Attempt to sit up. Sustain the contraction.

P10. Legs Thrust
Stand in doorway, legs bent, palms of hands overhead on door frame. Keeping arms straight, try to straighten legs.

P11. Side Foot Raise Against Wall
Stand beside a wall. Raise straight leg and press side of foot against wall. Turn round and repeat with other foot and leg.

P12. Heel Raise Against Wall
Stand with back to wall. Raise right heel against wall and try to flex further. Repeat bending left leg.

6.

Programme for Sitting Exercises

A head-to-toes isometric contraction programme may be performed while you are sitting on a chair (and even while lying in bed). Such a programme may have value for some elderly people, for convalescents, and for the disabled. A doctor's approval should be sought. People with weak hearts or high blood pressure should not perform the contractions.

Sports and body-training systems are often unsuitable for people in late middle-age and older, especially if they have neglected to take vigorous exercise for many years. There are problems of performance. If competition is involved, the older person may feel self-conscious or left out. The activities may be too demanding on the body. Isometric contractions are simple to perform – literally as simple as pressing two hands together. And they can be performed while sitting, thus conserving energy.

Conserving energy is helpful to the convalescent. Disabled people, confined to a wheelchair, should be able to adapt isometric exercises for their particular needs. Some disabled people become extremely strong and successful in sports and games, as the international 'Wheelchair Olympics' demonstrates.

A table chair to sit on is the most practical, since the held positions for isometric contractions usually require a straight back (though not rigidly straight) with head and back in poised line.

Instructions for Practice
General rules for practice were given in Chapter 2. The following points are worth noting again as they apply to the practice of the programme of sitting exercises.

Breathing

Take a deep but *comfortable* breath before starting the contraction. Feel as though air is going down to your abdomen as well as expanding your chest. Breathe in and out through your nostrils unless they are blocked or the special nature of an exercise requires mouth breathing. Most people will find that if a deep breath is taken the air can be released slowly from the lungs during a contraction lasting eight to ten seconds. A quick breath may then be taken and released slowly until the contraction is completed. Some people will experience no difficulty in exhaling during the whole of a contraction lasting fifteen seconds. The important thing is to avoid discomfort or strain in your breathing. Take an extra breath if you really need it, but remember that unnecessary inhalations disrupt momentarily the steadiness of your pressure.

Force and Duration of Contraction

Category A (moderate strength requirements). Elderly people and convalescents will fall into this category. Begin by sustaining each contraction for five seconds (a slow count of one, two, three, four, five). Add one second to the duration of each contraction at the end of each week until the duration of each contraction is ten seconds.

Start by exerting firm pressure without straining: about two-thirds of your maximum strength. Increase gradually until in about two weeks you are exerting strong pressure without straining, that is, about three-quarters of your maximum strength.

Category B (standard strength requirements). Begin by sustaining each contraction for six seconds (a slow count of one, two, three, four, five, six). Add one second per week until the duration of each contraction is twelve seconds. Exert power pressure, that is, about ninety per cent of your maximum strength.

Category C (maximum strength requirements). Begin by sustaining each contraction for nine seconds. Add one second per week until the duration of each contraction is fifteen seconds. Exert maximum pressure.

All categories should avoid muscle strain. Do not start with a sudden jerk. Apply steady pressure.

Elderly persons and convalescents should commence with Category A practice and elderly persons should stay in this category. Convalescents, as they return to health, should move into Category B, and when fully strong they may move to other programmes. Category C (maximum strength requirements) as applied to the sitting contractions will only be suitable for certain disabled persons aiming for great strength for sports and games. It will not require great imagination to adapt some of the exercises given in earlier programmes to their use. If in any doubt about the suitability of any exercise, you should always seek a doctor's advice.

S1ABC. Neck Contractions
The neck contractions given as the opening exercises in the programmes for both men and women can be performed while seated. For a description see M1A, M1B and M1C in the programme for men.

Your frontal, back and side neck muscles are strengthened, toned and rounded out by (A) pressing your head forward against counter pressure from your hands clasped on your forehead, by (B) pressing your head backward against your hands clasped across the back of your head, and by (C) pressing your head first to one side and then to the other side while preventing any movement by pressing the palm of your hand against the side of your head above the ear. (See illustrations M1A, W1B and M1C.)

If you have a chair with a high back that goes up to the top of your head or higher you can contract the muscles at the back of your neck by pressing your head back against it.

Another method is to fold a large handkerchief and pull it taut across your forehead, with your elbows raised out to the sides. To contract the frontal neck muscles, press your head forward and at the same time pull backward on the ends of a handkerchief. The handkerchief may also be pulled taut across the back of your head. The rear neck muscles are then contracted by pushing backward with your head and pulling forward on the handkerchief.

S2. Chair Shrug
This has been described and illustrated in the programme for muscle power. There is no reason why the elderly or convalescent person may not perform it, though the amount of muscular effort put into it should not match that of the sportsman or athlete.

You reach down and take a firm grip on each side of the seat of your chair. You need a good grip and not only the tips of your fingers. Some people may find that they need to place a cushion on the chair seat; as you sit up straight and grip the seat of the chair your arms should be straight. A straight-backed table chair is required for this exercise, and is, indeed, best for most exercises in the programme.

Take a deep breath then TRY TO SHRUG YOUR SHOULDERS UP TO YOUR EARS. Your straight arms and your grip on the chair seat will prevent any movement, but the image of a shrug should be in your mind. The effect of the attempted shrug is to produce a contraction across your shoulders. (See P2 for illustration.)

S3. Bent Arms Press In

The Press In with your hands clasped in front of your chest may be performed easily while you are sitting up straight in a chair. It has been described and illustrated in the programme for men M2. Bring the palms of your hands together before your chest in such a way that your upper and lower arms form right angles AND YOUR ELBOWS ARE HELD OUT WIDE. Take a deep breath, expanding and raising your chest, then PRESS YOUR HANDS TOGETHER STRONGLY. Neither arm should give way in the contest of strength. A static contraction will be produced in the muscles of your arms, shoulders and chest. (See M2 for illustration.)

S4. Bent Arms Pull Apart

Sit up straight, your knees a little apart and the soles of your feet flat on the floor. Now flex your left and right arms so that each forms a right angle between its upper and lower parts and lock your hands together directly in front of your chest by curling the fingers and thumbs of one hand firmly into those of the other hand.

Take a deep breath, then without moving your body or legs, TRY TO PULL YOUR HANDS APART.

This exercise will strengthen your rear upper arms, your upper back and your grip. (See M3 for illustration.)

S5. Fingers and Grip Strengthening

It is important that the elderly person or convalescent should retain adequate strength in the hands. Perform daily the finger and grip strengthening exercises described in the programmes for men and for women. These consist, first, of spreading your fingers and thumbs and pressing them down on a table top and, second, of squeezing your fists tightly or squeezing a small hard ball. Little breaths may be taken during the contraction.

S6. Table Press Up

Sit upright about thirty centimetres from a heavy table. Place the palms of your hands *below* the table top at shoulders' width. The seat should be the right height to produce right angles between your upper and lower arms, or close to it.

Take a deep breath then PRESS UP WITH BOTH HANDS AS THOUGH TRYING TO LIFT THE TABLE. During the contraction your back should be upright and you should look straight ahead.

The Table Press Up strengthens your hands, wrists, forearms, and upper arms. The chief muscles involved are those of the front upper arm which flex the arm. (See P6A for illustration.)

S7. Table Press Down

Continue to sit upright about thirty centimetres from a heavy table. Place the palms of your hands flat *on* the table top at shoulders' width. Again keep your upper arms in against your sides.

Keeping your back and head in a straight line, take a deep breath then PUSH DOWN HARD WITH BOTH HANDS.

This time the chief muscles contracted are those at the rear of the upper arms responsible for extending the arms. The hands, wrists, forearms and upper back also benefit. (See P6B for illustration.)

S8. Abdominal Retraction

Sit up straight with your knees and feet spread comfortably apart and the soles of your feet flat on the floor. Place the palm of your right hand on top of your right thigh a little above your knee and place the palm of your left hand on top of your left thigh a little above your knee.

Breathe out. On completing a full exhalation, DRAW BACK YOUR ABDOMINAL WALL TOWARDS YOUR SPINE, creating a hollow. A deep retraction is aided by rounding your back slightly and leaning forward slightly from the waist. HOLD THE RETRACTION FOR FIVE OR SIX SECONDS before releasing the abdominal wall and breathing in. Keep your breathing in suspension during the retraction; if you attempt to take an in-breath the muscles will recoil outwards. (See M9A for illustration.)

S9. Front of Thighs Contraction

We complete the programme of isometric exercises to be

performed when seated with two sets of contractions for the legs. Each leg is contracted separately and the other leg acts as an unyielding resistance.

Sit upright with your knees and feet a little apart and the soles of your feet flat on the floor. Raise your right foot and tuck its instep in against the back of your lower left leg.

Take a deep breath then TRY TO STRAIGHTEN YOUR RIGHT LEG. Keep your body upright and relaxed and localize all effort in your right leg. Rest a few moments then tuck your left instep behind your right calf, the sole of your right foot being flat on the floor. Take a deep breath then TRY TO STRAIGHTEN YOUR LEFT LEG. Your upper body should stay relaxed and unmoving.

This contraction works mainly the extensors of the thighs, frontal muscles of the upper legs. Your ankle and your knee joints are strengthened.

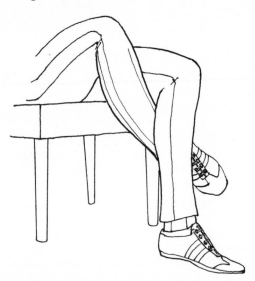

S10. Rear of Thighs Contraction

In the preceding pair of contractions you blocked the extension of your bent leg. Now you block an attempt to flex each leg.

Sit upright with your knees and feet a little apart and the soles of your feet flat on the floor. Raise your right foot and press the back of your ankle in against the front of your lower left leg just above your shin.

Take a deep breath then PULL YOUR RIGHT FOOT TOWARDS YOU. Keep your upper body upright and relaxed and localize all effort in your right leg. Rest a few moments, having returned the sole of your right foot to the floor. Raise your left foot and place the back of your ankle in against the front of your lower right leg just above your shin. Take a deep breath then PULL YOUR LEFT FOOT TOWARDS YOU. Your lower right leg will block the attempted flexion of your left leg.

The chief muscles exercised are those at the rear of the upper leg, which flex the leg.

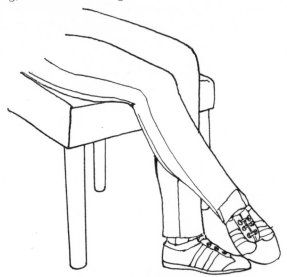

SUMMARY OF PROGRAMME OF SITTING EXERCISES

To be consulted as a rapid reminder of the programme only after correct performance of each exercise in every detail has been memorized.

S1ABC. Neck Contractions
A. Press head forward against clasped hands on forehead.
B. Press head back against clasped hands.
C. Press head to side against hand – first right side then left side.

S2. Chair Shrug
Sit upright and grip chair seat. Try to shrug shoulders.

S3. Bent Arms Press In
Press hands together in front of chest.

S4. Bent Arms Pull Apart
Lock hands in front of chest. Try to pull them apart.

S5. Fingers and Grip Strengthening
Press spread fingers and thumb down on table top. Squeeze a small hard ball or make tight fists.

S6. Table Press Up
Place hands under table. Press up.

S7. Table Press Down
Place hands flat on table top. Press down.

S8. Abdominal Retraction
Exhale fully. Draw back abdominal wall. Sustain the retraction.

S9. Front of Thighs Contraction
Tuck right instep behind left calf. Try to straighten right leg. Left instep behind right calf. Try to straighten left leg.

S10. Rear of Thighs Contraction
Back of right ankle above left shin. Pull right foot towards you. Back of left ankle above right shin. Pull left foot towards you.

7.

Programme of Exercises in Bed

Because of its economy of energy expenditure and indeed its total absence of movement, isometrics is an excellent exercise system for people confined to bed, the disabled, the blind, and the convalescent. Hospital physiotherapists included static contractions in their work with patients.

The fit and well may see some advantage in trying occasionally the following programme of isometric exercises that can be performed lying in bed, especially on a cold winter's morning. It will bring blood and life to the muscles of the whole body.

If you are confined to bed through illness or injury, it almost goes without saying that commonsense and caution should be used in the use of isometric contractions. Permission to use the exercises should be obtained from your doctor. People with heart disease or high blood pressure should not perform these contractions. Injured parts should not be exercised, unless with the permission of a doctor or a physiotherapist. On the other hand, there will be people for whom the following programme in whole or in part is a means of building and maintaining good tone and adequate strength in muscles likely to become flabby and weak.

Instructions for Practice
General rules for practice were given in Chapter 2. The following points should be noted as they apply to practice of the programme of exercises in bed.

Breathing
Take a deep but *comfortable* breath before starting the contraction. Feel as though air is going down to your abdomen as well as expanding your chest. Breathe in and out

through your nostrils unless they are blocked or the special nature of an exercise requires mouth breathing. Most people will find that if a deep breath is taken the air can be released slowly from the lungs during a contraction lasting up to ten seconds. The important thing is to avoid discomfort of strain in your breathing. Take an extra breath if you really need it, but remember that unnecessary inhalations disrupt momentarily the steadiness of your pressure.

Force and Duration of Contraction
Here we are only concerned with persons with moderate strength requirements. Begin by sustaining each contraction for five seconds (a slow count of one, two, three, four, five). Add one second to the duration of each contraction at the end of each week until the duration of each contraction is ten seconds.

Start by exerting firm pressure without straining – about two-thirds of your maximum strength. Increase gradually until in about two weeks you are exerting strong pressure without straining – about three-quarters of your maximum strength.

To avoid muscle strain, do not start with a sudden jerk. Always apply steady pressure.

B1. Neck Contractions
Your neck muscles can be strengthened, firmed, toned and contoured without your raising your head from your bed-pillow.

Lie flat on your back on the bed with your legs extended together. Breathe in and PRESS YOUR HEAD BACK HARD ON THE PILLOW. Rest a few moments. Turn onto your right side and PRESS THE RIGHT SIDE OF YOUR HEAD HARD ON THE PILLOW. Rest a few moments. Turn onto your chest and abdomen. Stretch your neck and tilt your forehead forward against the pillow. Breathe in then PRESS YOUR FOREHEAD DOWN HARD ON THE PILLOW. Rest a few moments. Turn onto your left side. Take a breath then PRESS THE LEFT SIDE OF YOUR HEAD HARD ON THE PILLOW.

If you prefer to perform these contractions – which strengthen the muscles at the back, sides and front of the neck – while lying flat on your back, then perform them using your hands for resistance as described and illustrated in the programme for men, M1A, M1B and M1C.

B2. Bent Arms Press In

Lie on your back with your legs extended. Clasp your hands above your chest so that your upper and your lower arms form right angles at your elbows.

Take a deep breath, expanding and raising your chest, then PRESS YOUR HANDS TOGETHER STRONGLY. (See M2 for illustration.) Your chest muscles, arms and shoulders will benefit.

Women wanting to firm and tone their busts should follow B2 with the following variation. Fully extend your arms overhead and bring together your palms and fingers as in the prayer position. Take a deep breath, expanding and raising your chest, then PRESS THE PALMS OF YOUR HANDS TOGETHER STRONGLY.

If a bedhead or wall does not permit an overhead extension of your arms, then extend your arms diagonally over your face.

This variation contracts and tones the upper fibres of the pectorals, the muscles which support the bust.

B3. Front Upper Arm Contraction

Lie flat on your back. Keeping your right arm in against your right side, raise your right lower arm to a vertical position, with the palm of your right hand facing your right shoulder. Reach across your diaphragm with your left arm and clasp your right palm with your left palm.

Take a deep breath, expanding and raising your chest, then TRY TO PRESS YOUR RIGHT HAND TOWARDS YOUR RIGHT SHOULDER BUT BLOCK ANY FLEXION WITH COUNTER PRESSURE FROM YOUR LEFT HAND. Rest a few moments then raise your left lower arm to a vertical position. TRY TO COMPLETE THE FLEXION OF YOUR LEFT ARM BUT BLOCK ANY MOVEMENT BY RESISTING WITH YOUR RIGHT HAND.

The arm flexing muscles at the fronts of your upper arms will contract, and your wrists and forearms will also benefit. (For an illustration of this exercise – in a standing posture – see M6A.)

B4. Rear Upper Arm Contraction

Now for the converse of B3. Instead of blocking an attempted flexion of each arm as in B3, you now block an attempted extension of each arm from a partly flexed position.

Lying flat on your back, bring up your right forearm to a vertical position, with your palm facing your right shoulder. Make a fist of your right hand. Reach across your body with your left hand and place your left palm against the back of your right fist.

Take a deep breath, expanding and raising your chest, then TRY TO STRAIGHTEN YOUR RIGHT ARM BUT PREVENT ANY MOVEMENT BY RESISTING WITH YOUR LEFT HAND. Rest a few moments, then reverse the roles of your arms and repeat the exercise. Take a deep breath, expanding and raising your chest, then ATTEMPT TO STRAIGHTEN YOUR LEFT ARM BUT BLOCK ANY MOVEMENT WITH COUNTER PRESSURE FROM YOUR RIGHT HAND.

The chief muscles exercised are those at the rear of the upper arms which extend your arms. Your wrists and your forearms also benefit. (See M6B for illustration.)

B5. Hand Strengthening
To build and maintain strength in your hands, SQUEEZE YOUR FISTS TIGHTLY. Squeeze first your right and, then squeeze your left hand, thus giving your full attention to each hand. You can take little breaths if required during each contraction. This exercise is worth repeating a few times each day. Your forearm muscles will benefit as well as your grip.

B6. Straight Arms Press Down
Lie flat on your back with your legs extended. Straighten your arms and place the palms of your hands flat on the bed about thirty centimetres away from either side of your body.

Without bending your arms, take a deep breath then PRESS DOWN STRONGLY WITH THE PALMS OF YOUR HANDS AND AT THE SAME TIME TIGHTEN YOUR ABDOMINAL MUSCLES.

This exercise achieves a double effect. Pressing down with your straight arms will contract the muscles of your upper back and at the same time you contract your abdominal muscles, firming and toning them.

B7. Lower Back Contraction
Turn over onto your chest and keep your legs extended together. Your arms should rest limply alongside either side of your body.

Take a breath then RAISE YOUR HEAD AND UPPER

BODY OFF THE BED AND SUSTAIN THE CONTRACTION. Without help from your arms you will not be able to lift very far, but the exercise will strengthen the muscles of your lower back.

B8. Abdominal Retraction

Turn over onto your chest and keep your legs extended together. Relax and exhale fully. Even when you feel you have fully emptied your lungs of air try to release a little more. Now DRAW IN YOUR ABDOMINAL WALL TOWARDS YOUR SPINE. If your exhalation has been thorough, a deep hollow will occur between your chest and your pelvis and eventually this will occur effortlessly or almost effortlessly. SUSTAIN THE ABDOMINAL RETRACTION for five or six seconds. Suspend your breathing during the retraction, as taking air into the lungs will cause the abdominal wall to move forward.

This yoga muscle control massages and tones the abdominal muscles and the internal organs which they support and protect. This control may be performed advantageously several times a day.

The Abdominal Retraction, performed in an upright posture, is illustrated following its description in the programme for men M9.

B9. Legs Raise

If there is nothing to preclude a more vigorous contraction of the abdomen, you can practise the legs raise described and illustrated in the programme for men, M10.

Lie flat on your back with your legs fully extended together. Take a breath then SLOWLY RAISE YOUR LEGS TOGETHER TO A HEIGHT OF THIRTY TO FORTY CENTIMETRES OFF THE BED. SUSTAIN THE CONTRACTION for the required number of seconds.

This exercise will strengthen the lower abdominal wall, firming and toning it.

B10. Knees Squeeze In

Sit on the bed with your knees drawn up and spread apart, and your ankles crossed. Cross your arms and place the palm of your right hand against the inside of your left knee and place the palm of your left hand against the inside of your right knee.

Take a deep breath and TRY TO BRING YOUR KNEES

TOGETHER BUT PREVENT ANY MOVEMENT WITH COUNTER PRESSURE OUTWARDS FROM YOUR HANDS.

The chief muscles benefitting are your legs, your arms and your chest.

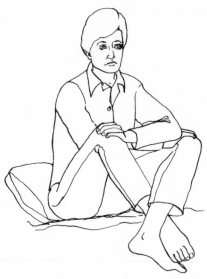

B11. Rear Upper Leg Contraction

Lie on your back with your legs extended together. Flex your legs to an angle of about forty-five degrees by raising your knees and drawing back your heels towards your buttocks.

Take a deep breath then PRESS YOUR FEET DOWN HARD ON THE BED. Have an image in your mind of pressing your feet down and towards you.

The bed resists an attempt to flex your legs, contracting the muscles of leg flexion at the rear of the upper legs. The hip joints and muscles also benefit.

B12. Lower Leg Contractions

Lie full length on your back on the bed with your legs fully extended. Raise your extended right leg to an angle of about forty-five degrees. Take a breath and then POINT YOUR RIGHT FOOT AND TOES AWAY FROM YOU. SUSTAIN THE CONTRACTION FOR THE REQUIRED NUMBER OF SECONDS. Without lowering your leg, breathe in and DRAW YOUR RIGHT FOOT AND TOES BACK TOWARDS YOU. SUSTAIN THE CONTRACTION FOR THE REQUIRED NUMBER OF

SECONDS. Lower your right leg slowly to the bed. Now raise your extended left leg to an angle of about forty-five degrees. Breathe in then POINT YOUR LEFT FOOT AND TOES AWAY FROM YOU. SUSTAIN THE CONTRACTION FOR THE REQUIRED NUMBER OF SECONDS. Keeping your leg raised, take a breath then DRAW YOUR LEFT FOOT AND TOES BACK TOWARDS YOU. SUSTAIN THE CONTRACTION FOR THE REQUIRED NUMBER OF SECONDS. Lower your left leg slowly to the bed.

Pointing your foot and toes will contract your calf muscles at the rear of your lower legs. Retracting your foot and toes will strengthen the fronts of your lower legs.

SUMMARY OF PROGRAMME OF BED EXERCISES

To be consulted as a rapid reminder of the programme only after correct performance of each exercise, in every detail, has been memorized.

B1. Neck Contractions
Press head back on the pillow. Press right side of head on the pillow. Press forehead down on the pillow. Press left side of head on the pillow.

B2. Bent Arms Press In
Press hands together in front of chest.

B3. Front Upper Arm Contraction
Flex right arm half-way at your side. Press left fist against right palm. Attempt complete flexion of right arm. Repeat for left arm.

B4. Rear Upper Arm Contraction
Flex right arm half-way at your side. Make fist of right hand.

Place palm of left hand under right fist. Press down with right fist and press up with left hand. Repeat for left arm.

B5. Hand Strengthening
Squeeze your fists tightly, first the right then the left.

B6. Straight Arms Press Down
Arms extended, press down with palms and tighten abdomen.

B7. Lower Back Contraction
Lying face down, raise head and upper body. Sustain contraction.

B8. Abdominal Retraction
Exhale fully. Draw back abdominal wall. Sustain the retraction.

B9. Legs Raise
Legs extended. Raise legs together diagonally and sustain contraction.

B10. Knees Squeeze In
Sit with knees drawn up and spread apart, ankles crossed. Palm of right hand against inside of left knee and left palm against inside of right knee. Try to bring knees together.

B11. Rear Upper Leg Contraction
Legs extended together. Partly flex legs. Press feet down and back.

B12. Lower Leg Contraction
Raise right leg diagonally. Point right foot and toes away from you. Sustain contraction. Draw foot back towards you and sustain contraction. Repeat with left leg.

8.

Exercises with a Partner

A number of the contractions described in the preceding programmes may be practised with a partner whose role is to supply the unyielding resistance. You return the favour by blocking attempted movements for him or her.

One advantage of exercising with a partner is that each person can make sure that the other person gives full concentration to each contraction and does not skip any exercises.

Another advantage is that an element of shared enjoyment and play enters your isometric programme. Children especially will find a shared programme a source of fun.

Isometrics for Children
Studies reveal that in the industrialized countries of the West there is not only widespread lack of exercise in adults but also increasingly in young people and children. Even when a child is more active than average in play and games, important muscles and muscle groups may not be exercised adequately. Isometric contractions are not difficult to perform and are adaptable to all degrees of available muscular strength. Three times a week is sufficient practice for children, as they are usually otherwise more active than their parents. Interest is added if they go through their programme with a partner of about equal strength, or if they make use of a belt or a folded towel.

Isometrics as Child's Play
If you want to see isometric contractions as child's play you have only to observe two chums engaged in rough and tumble fun. They will push and pull, press and squeeze – and if they

are of about equal strength you will see a number of static (isometric) contractions in the space of a few minutes. Here are some examples: pushing hands together; gripping wrists or locking hands to have a pulling contest; tug-of-war with a belt or rope; wrist wrestling; encircling head with arms and the attempt to get free; standing back to back with interlocked arms and bending forward to lift the other person onto your back (he or she then lifts you); bear hugs; and so on.

Look over the exercises given in the preceding programmes and you will see how in many cases a partner could provide the resistance.

Neck Contractions

In the neck contractions exercises a partner rather than your own hands could provide unyielding opposition to a head movement. Thus A stands behind B, who sits upright on a chair. A clasps his hands across B's forehead. B presses his head forward strongly while A prevents any movement by pulling back with his hands. Continue for the sides of the neck and the back of the neck.

Arm Exercises

A partner can block attempts to flex the arms or to extend them with the held positions similar to those described for contracting the front upper arms and the rear upper arms in exercises M6A and M6B. With a partner, an attempt can be made (and blocked) to bend further or to straighten both arms at the same time and not each arm separately as has to be done when your other arm provides the resistance.

The extensors of the arm, at the rear of the upper arm, are neglected muscles in most sedentary male workers and is often seen to be loose and flabby in middle-aged women wearing short-sleeved dresses. Here is a very effective exercise to strengthen, firm, tone and shape the rear upper arms. It has not been given earlier.

Sit upright. Flex your arms fully, lifting your elbows high with your hands behind your neck and your wrists almost touching your ears. The palms of your hands should face upward. Your partner blocks any movement as you try to straighten your arms overhead. The roles are then reversed and the exercise repeated.

To perform this exercise without a partner, contract first the right arm, blocking the extension of the arm by holding down your right hand with your left hand. Repeat, pressing down with your right hand on your left hand while you try to straighten your left arm.

Yet another version is to hold a belt or a folded towel taut between your hands so that it is held vertically down the central line of your back. In this case the palms of your hands may face the back of your neck (upper hand) and your lower back (lower hand). Again you should contract first your right arm and then your left arm.

Sit-ups and Leg-raises

Attempts at sit-ups or leg-raises can be blocked by pressure from a partner's hands. Similarly, attempts to raise the upper body while lying face down may be checked by the partner so as to contract the lower back.

If the partners sit on the floor facing each other, they can flex their legs and push the soles of their feet together in a leg-pushing contest. This exercises the front muscles of the thighs that straighten the partly flexed legs.

The flexor muscles at the rear of the upper legs can be exercised very effectively as follows. A lies on his stomach on the floor. Keeping his legs together, he brings up his lower legs to a vertical position of half-way flexion. B grips A's heels. A tries to complete the flexion of both legs but is prevented from doing so by B pulling back on A's heels. A then provides the resistance for B to perform the same contraction for the biceps of the thighs.

Feet Retraction and Pointing

In feet retracting and feet pointing, as described in M12 and in W10, a partner can grip the foot and ensure a strong contraction of the front lower legs and the calf muscles.

From what I have written above, it should be clear that a head-to-toes programme of isometric exercises can be shared advantageously by two people.

9.

Isometrics for the Face

Most people are aware of the importance of facial appearance, but comparatively few people are aware that the facial muscles respond well to direct exercise just as readily as those of say the arms or the legs. Contractions of the face muscles take much less effort than those for other parts of the body. You just pull a few faces of the kind men do when they shave.

I give a full guide to this neglected aspect of human exercise in my book *New Faces. Simple Facial Exercises to Keep You Looking Young*. Here I will describe two effective static facial contractions. Together they exercise most of the muscles of the face and should convince the newcomer of the value of facial exercise.

Even people who are aware of the need for regular planned exercise of their bodies mostly tend to neglect facial exercise simply because there is widespread ignorance about it. The reactions of the press to publication of *New Faces* was that here was a surprising novelty. Yet, when you think about it, is obvious that if we are going to exercise our muscles we should give attention to those muscles most open to the gaze of other people and those muscles whose contours and condition determine how other people read our characters and react to us. These intricate muscles reflect intimately our states of mind and markedly show evidence of civilized stresses and strains.

Like any other muscles, those of the face respond to exercise by becoming stronger, firmer, and improved in tone and shape. A healthy face is the foundation of a beautiful face in a woman and a handsome face in a man. Face exercises feed the tissues with blood, improve the complexion, and mould the face on more youthful lines. They smooth out wrinkles. They make the face more mobile and add life to the features. They promote a sense of well-being and self-confidence.

A few minutes exercise each day can lift years from facial appearance. In *New Faces* I give both isometric and isotonic exercises for the muscles of the face and the neck. Here are two isometric contractions which should demonstrate to you how valuable facial exercise can be.

Contraction of the Platysma

The platysma is the largest facial muscle: broad and flat, it extends from the cheeks, jaw and mouth down to the chest. It pulls down the corners of the mouth and maintains the contours of the neck.

Sit or stand with your head back in a straight vertical line. Breathe out for two or three seconds. Now bring your teeth together and pull down the corners of your mouth as far as they will go. The platysma will contract from your cheeks to your chest. Sustain the contraction for six seconds. Gazing at your reflection in a mirror as you exercise your face will aid concentration and performance. Release the contraction and relax and breathe normally for half a minute or so. Then repeat the facial contraction.

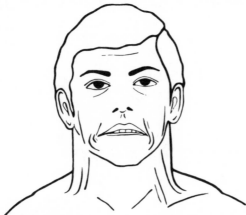

The Face of a Lion

This second exercise is valuable because it exercises most of the face. Once again we borrow from the postures of Hatha Yoga. The Face of a Lion Posture complements the preceding Contraction of the Platysma by lifting the face muscles and imparting a feeling of expansive well-being. The muscles of the face are toned, firmed, and made more mobile. A nourishing flow of blood is directed to the neck, the larynx, and the face. It is one of the earliest examples of an isometric contraction exercise. In yoga the whole of the body participates in the contraction and this approach adds to the effectiveness of the exercise.

The yoga method is to kneel with your knees together and to sit on the inner edges of your upturned feet. Place the palm of your right hand on your right thigh with the tips of your fingers a little above your right knee and place your left palm similarly on your left thigh. Your head and back should be in a poised vertical line.

An alternative position for people not wishing to adopt the traditional yoga posture is to sit erect on a straight-backed chair, with the palms of your hands on your thighs as described above.

Breathe out. Open your mouth as wide as possible and protrude your tontue out and down as far as possible. At the same time expand your face outwards in all parts and open your eyes wide. You should feel as though your face is radiating energy. As you expand your face muscles, straighten your arms and tense your whole body. Sustain the contraction for six seconds, with your breathing suspended. The total effect is invigorating and life-enhancing. Following the contraction, let go fully and breathe normally for half a minute or so. Then repeat the contraction.

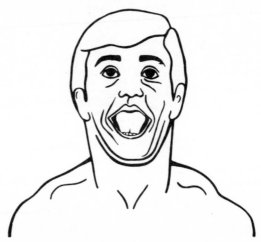

It is no exaggeration to say that facial exercises influence your state of mind as well as bringing health to the muscles. They break up and discourage tensions. Exercising the face helps dissolve mask-like rigidity of the kind one sees in emotionally repressed individuals. And for everyone it promotes increased awareness of the subtle and fleeting moods of the psyche, which is a form of greater self-knowledge.

10.

Total Fitness

It is important to understand that no exercise method fulfils your total fitness needs. Each emphasizes one or more aspects of fitness but misses out other aspects. Jogging, running, cycling, and brisk movement calisthenics put the emphasis on cardio-vascular fitness: through sustained muscle movements they stimulate the heart, the circulation, and the breathing. This is muscle endurance exercise. Yoga is unrivalled for achieving suppleness and joint flexibility, relaxation, body-mind integration and equanimity. Training with weights is a clear example of exercise which aims at muscle strength and tone. So is isometrics.

All these fitness aims are valuable, but each system mentioned leaves something out of the fitness picture. This applies to isometrics, in which the advantages of static contractions has to be weighed against their failure to exercise joints and muscles over their range of movement or to other than mildly stimulate the heart and the lungs. It is a fact of life that in exercise systems you cannot have everything. But if you are aware of what is lacking in your fitness training, then it is a simple matter to bring in the missing factors.

Strength and endurance are not the same thing. Muscle strength enables you to lift, pull, push, or otherwise move heavy loads for short periods. Muscle endurance enables you to be active for a long time. Weight-lifters train for great strength: for an explosive effort lasting only a few seconds. The professional boxer trains for endurance: to last perhaps fifteen three-minute rounds of activity. Isometrics, like training with weights, is primarily a strength builder. It will add something to endurance, but to complete your total fitness picture you should add direct endurance exercise of some kind. It will give you end-of-the-day energy and will strengthen your heart. Endurance exercise strengthens the heart in two ways: by improving the quality of its muscle and by increasing its efficiency.

You may already take active exercise – in your job or by walking, jogging, cycling, swimming, or whatever. But if you don't, even a little attention to this side of fitness-building and fitness-maintaining will pay dividends.

The human body needs regular movement exercise. If your daily life does not incorporate it adequately, then you should include at least ten minutes brisk continuous activity on alternate days. This can involve any exercise which sets your heart beating faster, your circulation speeding up, and your lungs expanding and contracting more vigorously. A gain in endurance fitness will augment your gain in strength and muscle tone from isometrics.

You can jog on one spot, though it soon becomes boring. Dancing in a lively manner to radio or record is an entertaining alternative. Fast keep-fit movements, brisk walking, swimming, cycling, skipping – anything that activates a higher heart rate without strain. Stop at any sign of distress, and if you have a health problem get your doctor's permission before you start exercising. Average fitness needs are met by about ten minutes activity, including (if necessary) rest intervals in which you continue mild movement.

If you are already experiencing the benefits of yoga practice you will not need to do anything further for attaining and maintaining flexibility, suppleness, relaxation, and psycho-physical harmony. Yoga goes well beyond the usual targets of fitness methods, aiming at nothing less than integration of the whole person – body, mind, and spirit. Several yoga exercises are included among the isometric contractions given in this book. Some of the postures (*asanas*) are difficult, but simplified Western adaptations are described in a large number of available books.

Your isometric programme should be practised daily for best results. Endurance fitness exercises may be performed on alternate days three times a week: either Monday, Wednesday, Friday or Tuesday, Thursday, Saturday. Whatever three days you select, use the other three days for flexibility fitness exercises. I confidently recommend yoga and, while arm and leg stretching and head and trunk twisting movements come second-best, they are certainly better than nothing.